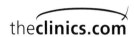

theclinics.com

# CRITICAL CARE NURSING CLINICS OF NORTH AMERICA

## Cardiopulmonary Resuscitation

GUEST EDITOR
Maria A. Smith, DSN, RN, CCRN

CONSULTING EDITOR
Suzanne S. Prevost, PhD, RN, CNAA

March 2005 • Volume 17 • Number 1

**SAUNDERS**

An Imprint of Elsevier, Inc.
PHILADELPHIA    LONDON    TORONTO    MONTREAL    SYDNEY    TOKYO

**W.B. SAUNDERS COMPANY**
*A Division of Elsevier Inc.*

The Curtis Center • Independence Square West • Philadelphia, Pennsylvania 19106

http://www.theclinics.com

**CRITICAL CARE NURSING CLINICS OF NORTH AMERICA**  Volume 17, Number 1
**March 2005**  ISSN 0899-5885
Editor: Maria Lorusso  ISBN 1-4160-2650-9

Reprints. For copies of 100 or more, of articles in this publication, please contact the Commercial Reprints Department, Elsevier Inc., 360 Park Avenue South, New York, New York 10010-1710. Tel. (212) 633-3813 Fax: (212) 462-1935 e-mail: reprints@elsevier.com

The ideas and opinions expressed in *Critical Care Nursing Clinics of North America* do not necessarily reflect those of the Publisher. The Publisher does not assume any responsibility for any injury and/ or damage to persons or property arising out of or related to any use of the material contained in this periodical. The reader is advised to check the appropriate medical literature and the product information currently provided by the manufacturer of each drug to be administered to verify the dosage, the method and duration of administration, or contraindications. It is the responsibility of the treating physician or other health care professional, relying on independent experience and knowledge of the patient, to determine drug dosages and the best treatment for the patient. Mention of any product in this issue should not be construed as endorsement by the contributors, editors, or the Publisher of the product or manufacturers' claims.

*Critical Care Nursing Clinics of North America* (ISSN 0899-5885) is published quarterly by W.B. Saunders Company. Corporate and editorial offices: The Curtis Center, Independence Square West, Philadelphia, PA 19106-3399. Accounting and circulation offices: 6277 Sea Harbor Drive, Orlando, FL 32887-4800. Periodicals postage paid at Orlando, FL 32862, and additional mailing offices. Subscription prices are $100.00 per year for US individuals, $164.00 per year for US institutions, $70.00 per year for US students and residents, $132.00 per year for Canadian individuals, $203.00 per year for Canadian institutions, $140.00 per year for international individuals, $203.00 per year for international institutions and $70.00 per year for Canadian and foreign students/residents. To receive student/resident rate, orders must be accompanied by name of affiliated institution, date of term, and the *signature* of program/residency coordinator on institution letterhead. Orders will be billed at individual rate until proof of status is received. Foreign air speed delivery is included in all *Clinics* subscription prices. All prices are subject to change without notice. POSTMASTER: Send address changes to *Critical Care Nursing Clinics of North America*, W.B. Saunders Company, Periodicals Fulfillment, Orlando, FL 32887-4800. **Customer Service: 1-800-654-2452 (US). From outside of the US, call 1-407-345-4000.**

*Critical Care Nursing Clinics of North America* is covered in *International Nursing Index, Nursing Citation Index, Cumulative Index to Nursing and Allied Health Literature, and RNdex Top 100.*

Printed in the United States of America.

## GOAL STATEMENT

The goal of *Critical Care Nursing Clinics of North America* is to keep practicing critical care nurses up to date with current critical care clinical practice by providing timely articles reviewing the state of the art in critical care.

## ACCREDITATION

The *Critical Care Nursing Clinics of North America* is planned and implemented in accordance with the Essential Areas and Policies of the Accreditation Council for Continuing Medical Education (ACCME) through the joint sponsorship of the University of Virginia School of Medicine and Elsevier. The University of Virginia School of Medicine is accredited by the ACCME to provide continuing medical education for physicians.

The University of Virginia School of Medicine designates this educational activity for a maximum of 60 category 1 credits per year, 15 category 1 credits per issue, toward the AMA Physician's Recognition Award. Each practitioner should claim only those credits that he/she actually spent in the activity. *NOTE: The American Nurses Credentialing Center (ANCC), and many State Boards accept AMA category 1 credit issued by an ACCME provider to maintain ANA certifications or licensure. 15 AMA category 1 credits are equivalent to 18 ANA contact hours.*

Category 1 credit can be earned by reading the text material, taking the CME examination online at http://www.theclinics.com/home/cme, and completing the evaluation. After taking the test, you will be required to review any and all incorrect answers. Following completion of the test and evaluation, your credit will be awarded and you may print your certificate.

## FACULTY DISCLOSURE

As a provider accredited by the Accreditation Council for Continuing Medical Education (ACCME), the Office of Continuing Medical Education of the University of Virginia School of Medicine must ensure balance, independence, objectivity, and scientific rigor in all its individually sponsored or jointly sponsored educational activities. All authors/editors participating in a sponsored activity are expected to disclose to the readers any significant financial interest or other relationship (1) with the manufacturer(s) of any commercial product(s) and/or provider(s) of commercial services discussed in an educational presentation and (2) with any commercial supporters of the activity (significant financial interest or other relationship can include such things as grants or research support, employee, consultant, stock holder, member of speakers bureau, etc.) The intent of this disclosure is not to prevent authors/editors with a significant financial or other relationship from writing an article, but rather to provide readers with information on which they can make their own judgments. It remains for the readers to determine whether the author's/editor's interest or relationships may influence the article with regard to exposition or conclusion.

*The authors/editors listed below have identified no professional or financial affiliations related to their presentation:*
Shirley W. Cantrell, PhD, RN; Angela P. Clark, PhD, RN, CNS, FAAN, FAHA; Sandra B. Dunbar, DSN, RN, FAAN; Nancy J. Finch, PhD, RN; Cathie E. Guzzetta, PhD, RN, CNS, FAAN, FAHA; Patricia Kunz Howard, PhD, RN, CEN; Kenya Kirkendoll, MSN, RN; Jonathan Langberg, MD; Marie Lasater, MSN, RN, CCRN; Rebecca E. Long; MS, RN, CCRN, CMSRN; Maria Lorusso, Acquisitions Editor; Theresa A. Meyers, MS, RN, CEN; Reverend Michael Norris; Marian C. O'Brien, MPH, RN; Suzanne Prevost, PhD, RN, CNAA, Consulting Editor; Nancy H. Romeiko, RN; Thomas D. Rone, BSN, RN, CCRN; Jenny L. Sauls, DSN, RN, C; Pamela P. Taylor, PhD, RN; Amy L. Valderrama, MSN, RN, APRN, BC; Wayne F. Voelmeck, MS, RN; Karen S. Ward, PhD, RN; and, Vicki L. Zeigler, MSN, RN.

*The author listed below has identified the following professional or financial affiliations:*
**Robert B. Leman, MD** has received grants from Medtronic, Guidant, and St. Jude.

*Disclosure of discussion of non-FDA approved uses for pharmaceutical products and/or medical devices:* The University of Virginia School of Medicine, as an ACCME provider, requires that all authors/editors identify and disclose any "off label" uses for pharmaceutical products and/or for medical devices. The University of Virginia School of Medicine recommends that each reader fully review all the available data on new products or procedures prior to instituting them with patients.

*All authors/editors who provided disclosures will not be discussing any off-label uses except:*
**Marie Lasater, MSN, RN, CCRN** will discuss the use of Meperidine to treat shivering.

*The authors/editors listed below have not provided disclosure or off-label information:*
Michael D. Aldridge, MSN, RN, CCRN; Margie Brown, RPh; Marcia A. Lankster, BSN, RN; Patti Loper, BA, RN, CHRN; Patty Nyquist-Heise, BSN, RN, CCRN; Maria A. Smith, DSN, RN, CCRN; and, Milton Stanhope Brasfield III, MD.

## TO ENROLL

To enroll in the Critical Care Clinics of North America Continuing Medical Education program, call customer service at 1-800-654-2452 or sign up online at **http://www.theclinics.com/home/cme**. The CME program is available to subscribers for an additional annual fee of $49.95.

# GUEST EDITOR

**MARIA A. SMITH, DSN, RN, CCRN,** Professor, School of Nursing, Middle Tennessee State University, Murfreesboro, Tennessee

# CONTRIBUTORS

**MICHAEL D. ALDRIDGE, MSN, RN, CCRN,** Pediatric Intensive Care Unit Nurse Educator/CNS Fellow, Children's Hospital of Austin, Austin, Texas

**MILTON STANHOPE BRASFIELD III, MD,** Pediatrician and Neonatal Advisor, Bryan W. Whitfield Memorial Hospital, Demopolis, Alabama

**MARGIE BROWN, RPh,** Director of Pharmacy Services, Bryan W. Whitfield Memorial Hospital, Demopolis, Alabama

**SHIRLEY W. CANTRELL, PhD, RN,** Associate Professor of Nursing, School of Nursing, Middle Tennessee State University, Murfreesboro, Tennessee

**ANGELA P. CLARK, PhD, RN, CNS, FAAN, FAHA,** Associate Professor of Nursing, University of Texas at Austin School of Nursing, Austin, Texas

**SANDRA B. DUNBAR, RN, DSN, FAAN,** Charles Howard Candler Professor, Nell Hodgson Woodruff School of Nursing, Emory University, Atlanta, Georgia

**NANCY J. FINCH, RN, PhD,** Clinical Assistant Professor of Nursing, College of Nursing, Medical University of South Carolina, Charleston, South Carolina

**CATHIE E. GUZZETTA, PHD, RN, HNC, FAAN,** Nursing Research Consultant, Children's Medical Center of Dallas, Dallas, Texas

**PATRICIA KUNZ HOWARD, PhD, RN, CEN,** Research Protocol Clinical Manager for Cardiovascular Nursing, University of Kentucky College of Nursing; and Staff Development Specialist, Emergency Department, University of Kentucky Hospital, Lexington, Kentucky

**KENYA KIRKENDOLL, RN, MSN,** Senior Research Nurse, Nell Hodgson Woodruff School of Nursing, Emory University, Atlanta, Georgia

**JONATHAN LANGBERG, MD,** Director, Section of Cardiac Electrophysiology, Emory University System of Healthcare, Atlanta, Georgia

**MARCIA A. LANKSTER, BSN, RN,** Director of Nursing, Bryan W. Whitfield Memorial Hospital, Demopolis, Alabama

**MARIE LASATER, RN, MSN, CCRN,** Staff Nurse, Neurosurgery ICU, Barnes Jewish Hospital, St. Louis, Missouri

**ROBERT B. LEMAN, MD,** Professor of Medicine and Co-Director, Adult Electrophysiology Laboratory, Department of Medicine, Medical University of South Carolina, Charleston, South Carolina

**REBECCA E. LONG, MS, RN, CCRN, CMSRN,** Clinical Nurse Specialist/Academic Educator, Veterans Affairs San Diego Healthcare System; and Clinical Lecturer, San Diego State University, San Diego, California

**PATTI LOPER, RN, BA, CHRN,** Emergency Department Nurse Liaison, Memorial Hospital, Colorado Springs, Colorado

**THERESA A. MEYERS, MS, BSN, RN, CEN,** Director, Emergency and Critical Care Services, Memorial Hospital, Colorado Springs, Colorado

**REVEREND MIKE NORRIS,** Staff Chaplain, Memorial Hospital, Colorado Springs, Colorado

**PATTY NYQUIST-HEISE, RN, BSN, CCRN,** Emergency Department Nurse Liaison, Memorial Hospital, Colorado Springs, Colorado

**MARIAN C. O'BRIEN, RN, MPH,** Research Project Manager, Nell Hodgson Woodruff School of Nursing, Emory University, Atlanta, Georgia

**NANCY ROMEIKO, RN,** Director, Pacemaker Clinic, The Emory Clinic, Atlanta, Georgia

**TOM RONE, BSN, RN, CCRN,** Patient Care Director, Intensive Care Unit, Middle Tennessee Medical Center, Murfreesboro, Tennessee

**JENNY L. SAULS, DSN, RN, C,** Associate Professor of Nursing, Middle Tennessee State University, Murfreesboro, Tennessee

**MARIA A. SMITH, DSN, RN, CCRN,** Professor, School of Nursing, Middle Tennessee State University, Murfreesboro, Tennessee

**PAMELA P. TAYLOR, PhD, RN, BC,** Director of Nursing, Critical Care Services, and Informatics, Middle Tennessee Medical Center; and Adjunct Faculty, School of Nursing, Middle Tennessee State University, Murfreesboro, Tennessee

**AMY L. VALDERRAMA, RN, MSN,** Doctoral Student, Nell Hodgson Woodruff School of Nursing, Emory University, Atlanta, Georgia

**WAYNE VOELMECK, MSN, RN,** Graduate Student, Cain Research Center, University of Texas at Austin School of Nursing, Austin, Texas

**KAREN S. WARD, PhD, RN,** Professor of Nursing and Coordinator of the RN/BSN Program, School of Nursing, Middle Tennessee State University, Murfreesboro, Tennessee

**VICKI L. ZEIGLER, RN, MSN,** Doctoral Candidate and Graduate Research Assistant, Texas Woman's University, College of Nursing, Denton, Texas

# CONTENTS

experience life-threatening events that involve the cardiovascular, cerebrovascular, and pulmonary systems. Early recognition of warning signs, activation of emergency medical systems within the community, basic cardiopulmonary resuscitation, early defibrillation, airway management, and intravenous medication administration are key factors in improving resuscitation outcomes.

## FORTHCOMING ISSUES

## RECENT ISSUES

---

### THE CLINICS ARE NOW AVAILABLE ONLINE!

Access your subscription at:
**www.theclinics.com**

---

ELSEVIER
SAUNDERS

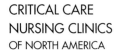

CRITICAL CARE
NURSING CLINICS
OF NORTH AMERICA

Crit Care Nurs Clin N Am 17 (2005) xv – xvi

Preface

# Cardiopulmonary Resuscitation

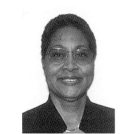

Maria A. Smith, DSN, RN, CCRN
*Guest Editor*

This issue of *Critical Care Nursing Clinics of North America* deals with the many facets of cardiopulmonary resuscitation (CPR). This closed-chest technique was first described in 1960 [1]. Since that time, research and technologic advances have enhanced the procedure with medications and electrical therapy. Since its inception, CPR has been used to save millions of lives. It is an essential ingredient in the fight against cardiovascular disease, the leading cause of death in the United States.

Cardiovascular disease accounts for the death of more Americans than any other disease. US citizens share this distinction with persons in Canada and Australia. More than one in five Americans has some form of cardiovascular disease. It is estimated that approximately 3 million Americans suffer occasional chest pain. Each year, at least 250,000 people die of myocardial infarctions before reaching a hospital. These deaths account for 29% of all deaths in the country [2]. These astonishing figures clearly demonstrate the need to continue evidence-based exploration of CPR to update nurses and other health care providers regarding this life-saving technique.

CPR has undergone continued revision and update, with the most recent recommendations occurring at the International Guidelines 2000 Conference on CPR and Emergency Cardiac Care. The article by Rone and Sauls presents an overview of the changes to the 1992 American Heart Association

guidelines. These evidenced-based changes fulfill the 1992 goal of producing guidelines that are international in scope. They pave the way for continued research in areas that extend from basic life support technique to advanced cardiac life support pharmacology.

Prevention of abrupt cardiac events is the preferable management mechanism for cardiovascular disease. As critical care nurses, we must focus on strategies to promote wellness in the population at large. When preventable causes are not abated by methods such as diet and exercise and heart disease results in the risk of sudden cardiac death, implantable devices can be used. Finch and Leman present plausible rationales based on research findings for the use of implantable cardioverter defibrillators in the prevention of potentially fatal arrhythmias. Even these devices are not without complications, however. O'Brien et al also present the implantable cardioverter defibrillators as primary and secondary prevention mechanisms for prevention of cardiac arrest; however, they also incorporate a review of storm, which is a complication of electrical intervention. It is important for nurses to be aware of the detrimental effects that even the best intervention devices can have when used for prevention.

Despite mechanical and electrical support, the heart may fail to initiate or maintain effective functioning without pharmacologic intervention. Medica-

doi:10.1016/j.ccell.2004.10.001

tion administration requires safe handling from the emergency department to the critical care environment. "High alert" medications used in the emergency department can carry death as a consequence of use errors. Brown explores safe medication practices from several perspectives, from dosages to incompatibilities. Medications administered in arrest situations are used to treat electrical and hemodynamic alterations that pose a threat to patient survival. Smith presents a review of vasopressors that have potent effects on the cardiovascular system. Vasopressors combined with CPR can promote return of hemodynamic stability.

Children are not immune to cardiac disease. These diseases may present minimal physical alterations or electrical dysfunctions that require pediatric advanced life support. Recognition of arrhythmias that cause hemodynamic compromise is imperative to pediatric management. Zeigler focuses pediatric management on electrical alterations that result in decreased cardiac output and poor perfusion. She presents electrocardiographic characteristics, clinical interventions, and nursing interventions for fast rhythms, slow rhythms, and collapse rhythms. The article by Lankster and Brasfield provides an update on pediatric advanced life support guidelines and presents an international perspective.

Despite aggressive efforts and implementation of pediatric advanced life support, the outcome for the pediatric client may be poor. This outcome affects all family members. Few studies have addressed post-resuscitation care. Cantrell and Ward examine physiologic management (ie, the sodium bicarbonate controversy) and emotional care (ie, separation from family and near-death experience). Clark et al present the advantages and disadvantages of family presence during CPR. Through case study format, they explain family presence from its history through implementation. Research is presented from various perspectives and you, the reader, are allowed an opportunity to draw your own conclusions based on the presented research.

CPR is only part of the total resuscitation event. It is important for nurses to have an accurate record of all occurrences during a CPR episode. Howard explores measures proposed in research to improve documentation during resuscitation, including the use of Utstein guidelines. Taylor presents handheld devices as expedient options to manage data during chaotic CPR episodes.

It is imperative that critical care nurses continue to maintain skill and clinical expertise in performing CPR. Long asserts that knowledge levels can be gained and maintained through the use of high-fidelity simulations. These simulations can facilitate transition of nurses from novices to experts. Nurses can use this knowledge to implement actions proposed by Lasater regarding thermoregulation during CPR. Through awareness of temperature measurement methods and limitations, nurses can combat the adverse consequences of hypothermia.

The goal of this issue is to update you on several of the multifaceted aspects of CPR. The authors have investigated these topics in an effort to present updates from education techniques to clinical practice.

### References

[1] Kouwenhoven WB, Jude JR, Knickerbocker GG. Closed-chest cardiac massage. JAMA 1960;173: 1064–7.
[2] US Department of Health and Human Services. Heart disease facts: Centers for Disease Control 2004. Available at: http://www.cdc.gov/nchs/fastats/heart.htm. Accessed September 30, 2004.

Maria A. Smith, DSN, RN, CCRN
*Professor, School of Nursing*
*Middle Tennessee State University*
*PO Box 81*
*Murfreesboro, TN 37132, USA*
*E-mail address:* massmith@mtsu.edu

ELSEVIER
SAUNDERS

Crit Care Nurs Clin N Am 17 (2005) 1 – 8

# Using Simulation to Teach Resuscitation: An Important Patient Safety Tool

Rebecca E. Long, MS, RN, CCRN, CMSRN[a,b,*]

[a]Veterans Affairs San Diego Healthcare System, Nursing 118, 3350 La Jolla Village Drive, San Diego, CA 92161, USA
[b]Department of Nursing, San Diego State University, San Diego, CA, USA

Knowledge, technical skills, and critical thinking. Methods to promote these crucial intellectual and physical nursing competencies are constantly being sought in a quest for an educational eureka [1,2]. Reports abound in the literature that reference the use of simulation to facilitate learning of many disciplines for decades. Early adopters of simulation include fields such as aviation, military, emergency medicine, and anesthesia. In health care, simulators have been used to train medical students, residents in surgery, obstetrics, radiology, and emergency medicine, and critical care nurses and respiratory technicians [3,4].

Seropian states in an article about simulation that "the belief that wisdom and clinical experience alone will produce safe, confident, and effective providers is likely fiction. So many nursing education programs are now using simulation to address issues of patient safety" [5]. Emergency situations present special challenges in fostering the ideal learning environment. Practicing on live patients is fraught with uncontrollable complexities [6]. Learning under duress in a situation in which mistakes may be critical to a patient's outcome is neither ideal nor in the best interest of patient safety.

This article highlights the author's and organization's experience with high-fidelity simulation and its use in facilitation of learning resuscitation scenarios. Simulation sessions with nursing students, experienced nurses, nurse anesthetists, physicians, and respiratory therapists are described. Novice to expert

principles—as they apply to resuscitation education by simulation—are highlighted. Detailed feedback obtained from nursing students is shared, as is general feedback from other disciplines. Finally, challenges for the future of simulation education are identified.

## Simulation in health care education

Simulation as an educational tool for teaching critical competencies during critical events has carved out a niche in the past several years. Affordability and improved quality of simulation models have contributed to its increased use [7]. Evolution of software programs, which interact with these simulators, has supported this growth. Maturation of the market to accept simulation as a viable educational tool is also responsible for this growth [3].

Simulation can be as simple as task and skill trainers, such as a rubber plate used for training with intravenous (IV) insertions. It can be as complex as a human-like mannequin complete with organ systems and internal software that provide physiologic responses. Fidelity is a term used to describe accuracy. Low fidelity relates to the static simulation tools, such as IV plates and catheter insertion models. High-fidelity simulation is the re-creation of a lifelike situation with maximal feedback and responsiveness. The perception of reality is stepped up a notch with the give-and-take potential of high-fidelity simulation.

Simulation can be used to teach critical incident nursing management (eg, emergency situations, such as pulmonary edema or cardiac tamponade) in nursing education. Nehring et al [1] described scenario

* Veterans Affairs San Diego Healthcare System, Nursing 118, 3350 La Jolla Village Drive, San Diego, CA 92161.
E-mail address: Rebecca.Long@med.va.gov

development for advanced medical surgical nursing, maternal and newborn care, and pediatric and nurse anesthesia courses. Simulation was used to provide a learner-centric model, which allowed faculty to evaluate and support students objectively in synthesizing knowledge and technical skills.

In the literature review, various terms, which are listed as follows, were noted to describe devices and systems used in simulation.

Body part simulation
Clinical simulation
Computerized models, computer simulation
Dynamic trainers, nondynamic trainers
Full-scale simulation
Haptics (using sense of touch)
High-fidelity simulation, low-fidelity simulation
High-level simulation, low-level simulation
Human patient simulator
Simulation
Simulator
Static simulation
Task trainers
Virtual reality

Simulation represents a human mannequin that has software located inside and is viewed by a personal computer. Software permits real-life scenarios to be constructed that represent patient management at the bedside. Models such as the SimMan (Laerdal, Stavanger, Norway) contain body parts similar to a human. Heart tones, murmurs, breath sounds, and bowel sounds can be programmed easily. Features include the ability to insert endotracheal tubes, chest tubes, nasogastric tubes, and IV catheters and view physiologic responses to interventions. Physiologic feedback to interventions with documentation by a computer and an audiovisual camera can be part of higher levels of simulation.

Many salient advantages of using high-fidelity simulation for education have been identified in the literature [7,8]. Key aspects of simulation training include the ability to train not only an individual but also a team. Leadership and communication skills can be observed and facilitated. Psychomotor skills can be learned and reinforced in a dynamic environment. Permission to make mistakes is unique to the simulation experience, and the ability to pause a scenario or skill for problem solving is optional. Identification of weaknesses of an individual during resuscitation, such as hesitancy to call for help or reliance on technology instead of physical assessment, can be identified with simulation [6]. "No industry in which human lives depend on the skilled performance of responsible operators has waited for unequivocal proof of the benefits of simulation before embracing it. ...neither should health care" is a persuasive statement that represents viewpoints from cheerleaders of simulation technology [9].

Various simulation models exist and have a wide range of prices (US $28,000–$200,000). In general, more expensive models are high fidelity and contain more sophisticated programming capabilities that may or may not be of value to the user(s). Creating virtual reality is the goal of the higher fidelity models. Several factors should be considered carefully before purchase of any model, as elucidated in Box 1 [1,5, 6,10–13].

---

**Box 1. System, equipment, and educational factors for consideration in development of simulation program**

*System*

General business plan
Goals of program
Location of equipment
Type of simulation desired
Cost: ongoing maintenance, fee structure
Faculty designation and availability
Ownership and governance of program
Information technology support for software installation and integration

*Equipment*

Degree of automation needed
Ease of use
Interactivity with computer system
Audio or visual capability
Cost: initial purchase
Software update availability
Vendor support
Portability

*Education*

Faculty training
Communication of program availability
Curriculum development: preprogrammed or created by faculty
Evaluation tool
Ongoing integration of evidence-based practice

## Experience of the San Diego Center for patient safety health care

### Simulation laboratory

High-fidelity simulation has been used at the Veterans Administration San Diego Health Care System and University of California at San Diego since August 2001. More than 400 hours of training using the SimMan have been offered to various health care practitioners, including nurses, physicians, and respiratory therapists. Simulation training is available for a fee to institutions and community agencies outside the Veterans Administration San Diego Health Care System and University of California at San Diego. Variable fees may include a wide range of services, including laboratory use, access to clinical instructors, technicians, and actors, scenario development, DVD archiving, video recording and editing, and use of general supplies. One hour of facility rental begins at $200. Development of scenarios is priced at a rate of $40 to $250 per hour depending on the discipline(s) involved.

### Nursing students in a medical surgical course

Approximately 36 San Diego State University nursing students participated in simulation training as part of their medical surgical course in the 2004 academic year. Simulation training occurred in groups of eight to ten individuals. Topics relevant to course content included anaphylaxis, acute coronary syndrome, addisonian crisis, tracheostomy with mucous plug (obstructed airway), cardiac tamponade, diabetic ketoacidosis, gastrointestinal bleeding, patient-controlled analgesia oversedation with respiratory arrest, pulmonary edema, and sepsis.

Scenario development integrated experiences to foster a "this really happened" element to the simulation experience. Approximately 60 minutes was required for the development of each scenario. Constructing realistic scenarios included writing objectives and integrating evidence-based signs and symptoms related to the clinical condition. Gathering supplies not stocked in the simulation laboratory required 30 minutes. A trial run of the eight scenarios with support personnel required an additional 2 hours.

Each student was assigned a disease or condition in advance and was required to complete a clinical worksheet. These worksheets contained items such as pathophysiology, signs and symptoms, complications, laboratory results, diagnostic tests, standard nursing care, and nursing diagnoses. Students were asked to complete the worksheet based on their fictional patient and include probable diagnostic results and potential complications. Students were asked to review any psychomotor skills that might be relevant. They were asked to keep their particular assignment confidential.

Sessions were 4 hours long. Students were asked to assume the primary nurse's place at the patient's side and respond to their scenario as it unfolded. Each scenario lasted approximately 20 minutes. A sample simulation scenario for anaphylaxis is presented in Box 2. Encouraging knowledge acquisition and critical thinking was a paramount goal. Assessment skills evaluated included differentiation of adventitious breath sounds, bowel sounds, and heart tones. Interventions necessitated the practice of various psychomotor skills. Demonstrations included insertion of urinary catheters, nasogastric tubes, oral airways, and disposable tracheostomy tubes. Other skills demonstrated included set-up of a chest tube drainage device, IV medication delivery, chest compressions, and ventilation with a bag/mask device.

Feedback from participants was overwhelmingly positive. Areas for improvement were obtained to facilitate future program growth (Table 1). A simple scale of 1 (not at all) to 10 (maximum possible) was used for a three-question evaluation tool. Results ranged from 9.3 to 9.6 (Table 2).

### Critical care nurses, physicians, nurse anesthetists, and respiratory therapists in a mock code blue

Real-time simulation education involved placing the simulation mannequin in an intensive care unit patient room and connecting it to a bedside monitor. An audiovisual camera was set up to capture the event. Members of the code team were informed that mock codes would be held in the near future. A code blue was called, and interdisciplinary team members arrived to find a simulation mannequin. The goal of this training was to emphasize proper implementation of the advanced cardiac life support (ACLS) tachyarrythmia protocol and observe communication and teamwork [14].

Several team members started to leave once they identified the situation not to be "real." They were asked to stay and conduct the resuscitation. In retrospect, to avoid some of the conflict experienced by asking team members to stay, additional reminders before these mock codes about the training sessions would have been helpful to foster collaboration.

Several key issues were identified related to lack of initial leadership and communication during the

---

**Box 2. Sample scenario for nursing students: anaphylaxis**

Level of learner: sophomore nursing students
Size of group: 8–10
Objectives: recognize anaphylaxis, state vital sign changes, review pertinent patient assessment, review what treatment to anticipate, state reason for each medication
Equipment/supplies needed: vital sign machine, IV pump, maintenance IV line with normal saline, secondary IV "piggyback" of piperacillin (Zosyn)
IV syringes, oral airway, bag/mask device, oxygen, nasal cannula, phone to call code "pretend"{ epinephrine, diphenahydramine, steroids)
Case scenario:
55-year-old man admitted for cellulitis. He has diabetes and peripheral vascular disease and smokes two packs of cigarettes per day. He has no known allergies. Shortly after starting IVPB piperacillin, patient complains of shortness of breath and appears flushed.

Course of simulation:

| *Patient characteristics* | *Expected nurse action* |
|---|---|
| Initial blood pressure 130/70; pulse, 72; respiration 18; temperature 99.8°F. SpO$_2$ 98 on room air, clear breath sounds | Administer IV piperacillin (demonstrate IV pump use) |
| "I can't catch my breath." Respiratory rate increases to 24, breath sounds wheezing, SpO$_2$ decrease to 88 | Assess breath sounds, count respiratory rate, observe work of breathing, note oxygen saturation |
| Blood pressure drops to 80 systolic, pulse increases to 120 | Note vital sign change, lower head of bed, administer oxygen 2L nasal cannula |
| "I'm itching all over" | Stops IV piperacillin and stop administration in current IV |
| Patient becomes stridorous | Demonstrate airway maintenance and bag/mask ventilation. State next steps: code blue/contact physician if nearby, administer epinephrine, antihistamines, consider steroids |
| RR decreases to 20, saturation to 94, breath sounds become clear "I feel less short of breath" | Administer IV fluids to maintain intravascular volume |
| Blood pressure increases to 110 systolic, heart rate decreases to 100 | Confirm allergy entered into patient record Educate patient regarding allergy and medication to avoid |

---

mock code. Mock codes are conducted routinely throughout nursing units but do not involve all disciplines. Experience has shown these mock codes to improve performance, and nurses believe they are helpful. One must question the reality and, more importantly, the effectiveness of the training of these single discipline sessions, however. Interdisciplinary teamwork is inherent and crucial in a resuscitation event. We have questioned whether the use of simulation could become standard to train all of our team members in bedside resuscitation (Barbara

Rose, RN, personal communication, 2004). We have not changed our training yet because of the staffing challenges involved with coordinating all disciplines concurrently but we plan to address this in the future.

*Physicians and nurses in advanced cardiac life support*

Approximately 60 ACLS participants were assigned to a 2-hour simulation session. Objectives included assessment of knowledge related to tachyar-

Table 1
Sample comments from nursing students regarding simulation experience

| Positive | Areas of improvement |
| --- | --- |
| "Very good to see what others are doing. . .feel like I learned from them" | "Didn't feel like I learned other patients as well as my own" |
| "I got a feel for an emergency situation, it seemed so real, and my heart was jumping out of my chest" | "Hard to concentrate for 4 hours, break it up" |
| "It gives you an idea of how fast things can go wrong and how I might respond under pressure" | "Try and speed up reactions. . ... some people just stood there in the beginning" |
| "This really tied a lot of things together for me". Actually seeing the patient respond was nice." | "I would like a little more information on the patients so I could be more prepared" |
| "I think this should be mandatory training every semester; I learned more today that I have in any class" | "Some things were a little confusing, because I didn't remember the diseases" |

rhythmia algorithms and demonstration of teamwork. Proper execution of tachyarrhythmia protocols was necessary, or the patient was programmed to deteriorate. For instance, when a wrong medication was given, the patient rapidly deteriorated and required further interventions. Critical thinking was assessed throughout the scenario by evaluating the actions of the individuals involved. Psychomotor skills demonstrated included application of pads and defibrillation, use of the automatic external defibrillator, chest compressions, delivery of medications in IV lines, intubation, and ventilation.

Table 2
Student Evaluation Tool n = 36

| Items | Responses |
| --- | --- |
| 1. Do you believe this experience enhanced the learning of your patient? | 9.5 |
| 2. Do you believe this enhanced your learning of the other patients? | 9.3 |
| 3. Do you believe this experience is relevant for the current course? | 9.6 |

Respond using a scale of 1–10. (1 = not at all; 10 = the maximum possible).

Participant feedback included statements regarding how realistic the simulation session was, including how responsive the mannequin (patient) was to interventions. Debriefing was a necessary component of these scenarios. Great concern was expressed for the patient, and several participants had a great deal of anxiety over their performance and its impact on the patient. This concern represented the affective domain of learning. Humor was used at the end of the session by programming a recognizable celebrity voice to thank the students for saving his life. The facilitator noted that having the responsiveness of the patient (mannequin) as part of the simulation experience resulted in sessions taking on a different flavor compared with previous sessions with a lower fidelity model (Karen Carroll, RN, personal communication, 2004).

## Novice to expert theory: lessons learned

The Dreyfus model of skill acquisition has value in applicability to a wide range of learners, both in experience and discipline [15]. Many of the behavioral and learning traits consistent with this model in various disciplines have been observed using simulation. Benner's classic work on novice to expert nurses has particular value in simulation education for nurses [16]. Novice, advanced beginner, competent, proficient, and expert traits were observed in the various groups in which simulation was used. When discussing learners in general in the psychological literature, Ericsson used the term "novice to champion" and noted that variations "are among the largest reproducible differences in performances observed for normal adults" [17]. Other work in experiential (practice-based) learning provides educators important information upon which to base simulation training [18,19]. Keeping the novice to expert theories as a foundation, training with simulation provides the ability to adapt the system to the type and level of learner.

### Novice and advanced beginner

Nursing students were judged to be novices. Recognition that complex scenarios would prove too difficult was important. Although a foundation of basic knowledge and skills was assumed to be present from earlier course and clinical work, a stressful situation can lead to a crumbling of ability in recall and performance. Much of the simulation literature emphasizes the importance of keeping the sessions real and lifelike. It was found to be helpful, however, when faculty paused the scenario to teach and add some humor when appropriate. The first few scenarios took longer than expected because of the pauses and students sometimes finding themselves "stuck." This could reflect lack of knowledge, disabled critical thinking, or performance anxiety. It is consistent with traits of a novice learner because they are rule based. Benner stated that because of the lack of experience of novices, they must be given rules to guide their performance [16]. Students were reminded to refer to the clinical worksheet that they had prepared for this type of patient (hopefully discovering some of the rules). This review often allowed students to proceed, but it did take more time. After this challenge was identified, more time was allotted for subsequent simulation sessions.

Keeping student performance expectations realistic is consistent with Benner's principles of not expecting novice learners to be able to judge the importance of various aspects of a scenario. In keeping with this principle, great care was taken to facilitate a positive and not punitive learning environment. Most scenarios were chosen to reflect current course content. Others were chosen to integrate technical skills, such as chest tube set-up. The more complex scenarios, such as acute coronary syndrome and cardiac tamponade, were assigned to students who had prior health care experience, such as emergency medical technician and anesthesia technician training. Because of their prior experience, it was known that they had experienced these situations several times and might be able to judge which aspects were meaningful. These traits, however, are more consistent with an advanced beginner.

Advanced beginners are known to have marginally acceptable performance and can extract meaningful components of a situation. Examples of this included a new graduate nurse taking ACLS for the first time. While implementing the ventricular tachycardia algorithm, it was unreasonable to expect this nurse to be able to set priorities of the arrest precisely. The nurse was not able to sort out the important and cast aside the unimportant. Ideally, a new graduate nurse would not be requested to serve as team leader for a resuscitation event until he or she demonstrated the ability to set priorities.

*Competent, proficient, and expert*

How does one offer the same scenario to learners with varied ranges of experience and disciplines? In reality, we know that any team that is convened in emergent situations typically has different disciplines and varied levels of experience. Replicating the challenging dynamic of this environment with simulation was the goal of the mock code training and the ACLS training. Unlike the protocols for nursing students, branching logic was used in the algorithms for these two groups. This type of event "reactivity" could result in the death of a patient if the correct interventions were not performed in a timely fashion.

In the ACLS training scenarios, participants included nurses from the new graduate level and nurses with several years of experience. They were deemed to possess traits consistent with novice, advanced beginner, competent, proficient, and expert levels. Physicians, medical students, and respiratory therapists had a similar wide range of experience.

A competent performer is able to distinguish relevancy. Giving a competent nurse practice in arranging multiple priorities is reasonable. This person may lack speed, but there is deliberate planning witnessed in his or her practice. During the ACLS training, the competent nurse was able to lead the group appropriately through resuscitation.

The proficient performer has an intuitive grasp of the scenarios based on a deeper understanding. They are able to see situations as wholes, which improves decision making. The proficient nurse is able to focus on a particular finding as important. Designing simulation scenarios with irrelevant findings for this learner is important to challenge the ability to apply knowledge and differentiate meaningful data. Simulation training can be ideal for this learner, who is often best taught with case studies. Validation of critical thinking via verbal explanations is important to support the proficient performer.

The expert practitioner is described as a hybrid who relies on practice and theoretical knowledge in decision making. They often interpret situations based on their gut and may have difficulty explaining the rationale. "Mature and practiced" reasoning is exhibited by the expert nurse [20]. It was noted in the mock code that several expert nurses in attendance were able to diagnose the situation quickly based on features that were less obvious to other nurses. This group of learners often uses analytic ability when they encounter unusual situations. A dynamic simulation environment with algorithms that require analytical thought and processing of the whole is valuable for the expert practitioner. An example is a patient who experienced cardiac tamponade on hospital day 4. Although overt signs and symptoms may not be present, when queried about potential causes, the expert cardiac surgery nurse may correlate the removal of pacemaker wires and resultant coronary artery displacement as a possible cause for the complication.

Deliberate practice is described as one of the key factors responsible for distinguishing the expert performer from others [17]. This statement would lead one to acknowledge the value of simulation in promoting simulation as a tool for resuscitation education. Skilled practitioners can work many years and yet not experience the wide array of emergency situations needed to maintain competency.

It is important to keep the range of learners, the skills of the facilitators, and the objectives in mind when designing simulation training sessions. Just as in other methods of education, there is no one-size-fits-all solution. Identical scenarios can be presented to different practitioners or teams by making a few adjustments in the scenario program. Titrating the knowledge required in a simulation scenario or editing a particular psychomotor skill can be accomplished relatively easily when conducting a scenario. This can be accomplished with specially designed scenarios or programs that already exist in high-fidelity simulators.

## Future challenges

Results of educational endeavors with simulation should be sufficient to support purchase and continued use. Unfortunately, nursing or medical research that documents the cost/benefit ratio of high-fidelity simulation as an educational intervention has been reported with less frequency and fervor than straightforward advantages and disadvantages. Although numerous anecdotal reports exist, well-constructed studies that examine these issues are important to validate. Ravert [21] reviewed quantitative studies related to simulation. Despite 513 references, only nine quantitative studies met the inclusion criteria. The review revealed that 75% of included studies showed positive effects of simulation on acquiring knowledge or skills.

It may be time to re-evaluate the gold standard for research as it relates to educational methods, however. In medical education research, Harden et al [22] noted that randomized controlled trials have been cast aside in favor of methods based on quality, utility, and strength of evidence. Educational researchers from other disciplines have long since abandoned the traditional randomized controlled trials [23]. Using randomized controlled trials requires informed consent, and randomization removes the choice of educational method from the participants. Harden questions, "How many adult learners would be prepared to pay for education services in which they were not able to choose the learning process?" The importance of evaluating the effectiveness of resuscitation education was discussed by the International Liaison Committee on Resuscitation at their 2002 symposium on education in resuscitation. In their report, they recommended a tool that accurately evaluates educational interventions "in providing the best skills acquisition and retention attainable" [24].

Proof of economic sustenance is also relevant in current fiscally challenging times. A business model that outsources a simulation laboratory experience to community venues may be more cost effective. Such a model offers a way for organizations without simulators to own devices and provide access to the community. This type of arrangement may result in $62,750 of net revenue per semester, as noted by Peteani [25]. This model included three clients purchasing a limited package that required the purchaser to supply its own curriculum and instructors.

## Summary

One must ask if existing methods of translating knowledge to practice, including clinical guidelines and textbooks alone, are adequate. Chamberlain [26] offers those of us concerned with outcomes of educational interventions (eg, simulation) the following perspective: "There are lessons to be learned from the history of resuscitation. Progress in all disciplines can be hastened if new ideas are welcomed but then evaluated critically; if old practices are not discarded until they can be replaced by others that are demonstrably better."

Despite a vast amount of literature available related to simulation, there must be continued exploration and elucidation of best practices of simulation as it relates to resuscitation education. Evaluation tools that measure educational outcomes of simulation education must be established. Economic evaluations of simulation purchase and use are important aspects of transitioning to this new technology. Simulation can offer fruitful development of critical thinking and psychomotor skills critical to effective resuscitation training. Individual and team performance can be assessed. Simulation programs can play an important role in promoting patient safety, and their role in this arena will continue to unfold.

## Acknowledgments

The author would like to thank Martha Shively, PhD, RN, and Kathleen Dunn, MS, RN, for thoughtful review of the manuscript. The author also would like to thank Matthew Weinger, MD, and Chris Rom, MD, for their assistance and support of the simulation program.

# References

[1] Nehring W, Lashley F, Ellis W. Critical incident nursing management using human patient simulators. Nurs Educ Perspect 2002;23(3):128–32.

[2] Del Bueno D. The cost of competence. Nurs Econ 2001;19:250–7.

[3] Issenberg S, McGaghie W, Hart I, et al. Simulation technology for health care professional skills training and assessment. JAMA 1999;282(9):861–6.

[4] Kapur P, Steadman R. Patient simulator competency testing: ready for takeoff? Anesth Analg 1998;86:1157–9.

[5] Seropian M, Brown K, Gavilanes J, et al. An approach to simulation program development. J Nurs Educ 2004;43(4):170–4.

[6] Hammond J, Bermann M, Chen B, et al. Incorporation of a computerized human simulator in critical care training: a preliminary report. J Trauma 1992;53(6):1064–7.

[7] Feingold C, Caluluce M, Kallen M. Computerized patient model and simulated clinical experiences: evaluation with baccalaureate nursing students. J Nurs Educ 2004;43(4):156–63.

[8] Rauen C. Using simulation to teach critical thinking skills: you can't just throw the book at them. Crit Care Nurs Clin North Am 2001;13(1):93–103.

[9] Gaba D. Improving anesthesiologists' performance by simulating reality. Anesthesiology 1992;76:491–4.

[10] Seropian M. General concepts in full scale simulation: getting started. Anesth Analg 2003;97(6):1695–705.

[11] Smith N. Simulation in anesthesia: the merits of large simulators versus small simulators. Curr Opin Anaesthesiol 2002;13:659–65.

[12] Seropian M, Brown K, Gavilanes J, et al. Simulation: not just a manikin. J Nurs Educ 2004;43(4):164–9.

[13] Rauen C. Simulation as a teaching strategy for nursing education and orientation in cardiac surgery. Crit Care Nurs 2004;24(3):46–51.

[14] Channing L. The tachycardias: overview of algorithm. In: Cummins RO, editor. ACLS provider manual. Dallas (TX): American Heart Association; 2001. p. 157–65.

[15] Dreyfus H, Dreyfus S, Athanasiou T. Mind over machine. New York: Free Press; 1986.

[16] Benner P. From novice to expert: excellence and power in clinical nursing practice. San Francisco: Addison-Wesley; 1984.

[17] Ericsson K, Krampe R, Tesche-Rome C. The role of deliberate practice in the acquisition of expert performance. Psychol Rev 1993;100:363–406.

[18] Zapp L. Use of multiple teaching strategies in the staff development setting. J Nurs Staff Dev 2001;17(4):206–12.

[19] Lighthall G, Barr J, Howard S, et al. Use of a fully simulated intensive care unit environment for critical event management training for internal medicine residents. Crit Care Med 2003;31(10):2437–43.

[20] Benner P. Becoming an expert nurse. Am J Nurs 1997;92(6):16BBB–DDD.

[21] Ravert P. An integrative review of computer-based simulation in the education process. Comput Inform Nurs 2002;20(5):203–8.

[22] Harden R, Grant J, Buckley G, et al. Best evidence medical education: Guide No. 1. Dundee: Association for the study of medical education in Europe; 1999.

[23] Prideaux D. Researching outcomes of educational interventions: a matter of design. BMJ 2002;324:126–7.

[24] Chamberlain D, Hazinski M. Education in resuscitation: an ILCOR symposium. Circulation 2003;108(20):2575–94.

[25] Peteani L. Enhancing clinical practice and education with high-fidelity human patient simulators. Nurs Educ 2004;29(1):25–30.

[26] Chamberlain D. Never quite there: a tale of resuscitation medicine. Clin Med 2003;3(6):575–7.

ELSEVIER
SAUNDERS

CRITICAL CARE
NURSING CLINICS
OF NORTH AMERICA

Crit Care Nurs Clin N Am 17 (2005) 9–16

# Implantable Cardioverter Defibrillator Storm: Nursing Care Issues for Patients and Families

Marian C. O'Brien, RN, MPH[a],*, Jonathan Langberg, MD[b],
Amy L. Valderrama, RN, MSN[a], Kenya Kirkendoll, RN, MSN[a],
Nancy Romeiko, RN[a], Sandra B. Dunbar, RN, DSN, FAAN[a]

[a]Nell Hodgson Woodruff School of Nursing, Emory University, 1520 Clifton Road NE, Atlanta, GA 30322, USA
[b]Section of Cardiac Electrophysiology, Emory University System of Healthcare, Emory Clinic, 1365 Clifton Road NE,
Atlanta, GA 30322, USA

The Multicenter Automatic Defibrillator Implantation Trial II published in May 2003, combined with evidence from other trials, led to increasingly widespread use of implantable cardioverter defibrillators (ICDs) for primary prevention of life-threatening arrhythmias in patients after myocardial infarction with a left ventricular ejection fraction of 30% or less [1]. This study showed a 31% survival benefit in patients who were randomly assigned to receive an ICD. More than 3 million patients in North America currently meet these criteria, with 400,000 more projected to meet them each year [2,3]. The rate of prophylactic ICD implantation is expected to continue rising as additional patient populations likely to benefit are identified. The SCD-HeFT Trial suggests that patients with nonischemic cardiomyopathy have improved survival with an ICD [4,5].

ICDs are small implanted pulse generators with circuitry that detects and records arrhythmic events 24 hours a day and delivers instantaneous therapy. The components are enclosed in a small titanium can [6] and are connected to one or more leads that sense electrical activity and serve as a conduit for therapy delivery. The ICD is programmed by clinicians to respond using bradycardia pacing, anti-tachycardia pacing, cardioversion ("light" shocks of 2–5 J), or defibrillation (15–40 J) when an arrhythmia is detected.

Biventricular ICDs are an important technologic and clinical advancement. They combine the function of conventional ICDs with the ability to pace the right and left ventricles simultaneously. In patients with congestive heart failure and intraventricular conduction delay (QRS width >120 msec), simultaneous pacing of both ventricles has been shown to improve hemodynamics, ejection fraction, and functional status [7]. Biventricular ICDs can improve quality of life and reduce the risk of cardiac arrest.

Increased implantation of ICDs and biventricular ICDs means more patients will likely experience shocks and, in some cases, present with defibrillation-related issues. One such issue is ICD storm, which is defined as a series of two or more ICD shocks (appropriately or inappropriately triggered) in succession within a 24-hour period. ICD storm occurs in 10% to 20% of patients [8,9] and is more likely in men [10]. ICD storm can occur anytime, but the peak incidence is 9 ± 12 months after implantation [11]. The clustering of shocks within a 24-hour period distinguishes ICD storm from multiple shock occurrences over longer periods of time. With more devices in use since the Multicenter Automatic Defibrillator Implantation Trial II, Defibrillators in Nonischemic Cardiomyopathy Treatment Evaluation [12], and Comparison of Medical Therapy, Pacing,

This work partially supported by funding from NIH NINR R01# NRO5187 Psychoeducational Intervention for ICD Patients.
* Corresponding author.
E-mail address: mcobrie@emory.edu (M.C. O'Brien).

and Defibrillation in Heart Failure studies [13], the number of patients at risk for ICD storm is increasing. Advances in technology, such as arrhythmia discriminators in dual chamber devices, which distinguish between supraventricular and ventricular arrhythmias, hopefully will reduce the occurrence of ICD storm through more sophisticated programming options [14]. The objective of this article is to provide an update for clinicians on the effects of ICD storm on patients and family members through literature review and interviews with patients who have experienced ICD storm.

## Factors associated with storm

To date there is no way to predict who will receive shocks from an ICD or when it will occur. Several studies have examined factors associated with ICD shocks in an effort to predict these events better. The Triggers of Ventricular Arrhythmias study included 1140 patients and found that New York Heart Association Class III heart failure and left ventricular ejection fraction <20% were independent risk factors for appropriate ICD shocks, ventricular tachycardia, and ventricular fibrillation [15]. The combination of New York Heart Association Class III and left ventricular ejection fraction <20% imparts a high risk for shocks. Factors associated with storm have not been well studied; however, approximately 30% of storm cases are triggered by atrial arrhythmias [16]. Inappropriate shocks occur in 14% of patients and may or may not be categorized as storm. It is more likely to occur in patients with pre-existing atrial arrhythmias, coexistent appropriate ICD therapy, and single-chamber ICDs [17].

## Causes of storm

Triggers of storm are varied and mostly unpredictable. It may happen when levels of anti-arrhythmic drugs are insufficient because of missed doses, there is a need for increased dose, or combined increased drug and device therapies are required because of progressive cardiomyopathy [6]. Storm also may occur when a supraventricular arrhythmia with rapid ventricular response is misinterpreted. Dual-chamber devices, which are being used more widely, are less likely to produce this problem because of arrhythmia discriminator technology. Electromagnetic interference or lead fracture also can cause storm [6]. Lead fracture causes false signals and inappropriate shocks and requires surgical revision. Hypokalemia, hypomagnesemia, and acute myocardial ischemia also may precipitate ICD storm [8]. In patients with biventricular ICDs, double counting of pacing spikes, which leads to electrical storm, is reported in 3% of patients [18].

The experience of ICD shock recently was linked to negative outcomes. Results of the Antiarrhythmias Versus Implantable Defibrillators trial revealed that the occurrence of storm for ventricular tachycardia or ventricular fibrillation is an independent marker for subsequent death in patients with ICDs, with a 5.4-fold increase in the risk of death in the first 3 months after storm [11]. The shock experience is also associated with lower quality of life [19], psychological distress [20], and increased depressive symptoms [21] and merits focused clinical attention.

## Storm cases

Six interviews with patients who had ICD storm—three with a low number of ICD storm shocks and three with a high number of ICD storm shocks—are presented to demonstrate common issues related to storm and highlight differences and similarities among participants in this sample. Interviews were conducted by phone after obtaining written informed consent and occurred between 2 and 12 months after the storm. None of the interview participants had biventricular ICDs. Some of the participants had storm more than once and were asked to think about the first time for the purpose of the interview.

### Case #1

A 36-year-old African-American man experienced an ICD storm while driving alone less than a week after his single-chamber ICD implant. He had a history of dilated cardiomyopathy with left ventricular ejection fraction of 20% and New York Heart Association Class II symptoms. When he received the first of the four storm shocks, he said he thought someone had hit him in the rear bumper. When he received the second shock and realized what was happening, he pulled the car off the road, at which point he received more subsequent shocks. He could feel and hear his heart beating but had never noticed having palpitations before. He tried to calm down by taking deep breaths, and then he rested for 10 to 15 minutes, drove home, and had a friend take him to the emergency room. He remembers wanting the device taken out initially, but he reports being glad that he has the ICD and wonders what would have happened to him without it.

He has had three isolated shocks since the storm and says it is not as bad when just one shock occurs. He was shocked while on a cruise and was sent home because of his health. He also was shocked once during sexual intercourse and abstained from intimate relations for approximately 6 months afterward. He avoids overexerting himself in an effort to prevent increasing his heart rate and triggering further shocks. Work and interacting with people helped him to cope psychologically with the storm episode. He says this is because he does not think about his heart when he is busy. He perceives that his family initially was overly protective but they have adjusted and are less protective. He recommends support groups for patients with ICDs or some kind of dialogue with others if a support group is not available.

*Case #2*

A 60-year-old African-American man with a history of coronary artery disease and a dual-chamber ICD was walking to meet friends to go fishing when he was shocked two times, 3 weeks after his implant. He had no warning but yelled immediately because it sounded like a "firecracker had gone off in [his] ear." He later was told that atrial fibrillation was the cause of the storm and that medication could prevent further occurrences. He had three isolated shocks before the storm experience: during sexual intercourse, after a minor automobile accident, and while walking. He thinks the shocks have reduced his daily activity level because he is fearful of receiving a shock from overexertion and heart rate increase. He says he has gained 32 pounds since the ICD implant because of his reduction in activity. He currently takes his medication daily as instructed because he was informed that the medication would have prevented the shocks. Family members have moved in with him, but he states that he would like to regain his independence from his family in the near future. He recently shared his ICD experience with another man who had been shocked after noticing that the man seemed worried, and they concluded that the defibrillator is "just doing what it's supposed to do" when it shocks them.

*Case #3*

A 63-year-old white man with a history of cardiac arrest and coronary artery disease had an ICD storm 1 week after implant. He was cutting his grass in the early evening when he received the first shock and went inside to lie down, at which time he was shocked again. He says he was "really surprised" and thought the shock was from the lawn mower at first. He called his cardiologist and went to the hospital via ambulance. His two shocks were 5 minutes apart, and he had no warning symptoms. He was informed later that atrial fibrillation triggered the ICD storm. Because he had angioplasty recently and had learned about damage to his heart from previous heart attacks, he knew that his heart was "in fragile condition." He described the shocks as intense and unpleasant but not painful.

The storm left him feeling stunned, and he compared the shock to a previous time when he broke his arm and had it set without sedation. He has had two isolated shocks since the storm but had a dizzy feeling before the isolated shocks. He felt like he was "walking on eggshells" for 3 to 4 days after the first isolated shock, but the next time it only took 1 to 2 hours to get rid of that feeling. After the storm experience, he altered plans to take a long driving trip and took a friend instead of going alone. He feels that the symptoms of rapid heart rate and dizziness are sufficient to warn him to get off the road, thereby allowing him to drive alone. He says that it is good to know that the ICD works and believes his outlook has improved because he knows the device can save his life. Having the device checked and reprogrammed was helpful immediately after the ICD storm. He was glad to know that the ICD programming change would prevent atrial fibrillation from causing shocks again and that the storm was not caused by deterioration of his cardiac status. As instructed by his cardiologist, he continued with his current diet, exercise program, and medications. His family was concerned about his health after the ICD storm, but the concern has lessened with time. Receiving information about the defibrillator was helpful and made him feel confident about his treatment.

*Case #4*

A 66-year-old white woman with a history of coronary artery disease and cardiomyopathy was in the bathroom when her ICD storm began. She states that it felt like a "mule kicking" but that she did not have any warning symptoms. She received a total of 25 consecutive shocks and states that she felt "really scared." Upon examination, she was told that her shocks were caused by atrial fibrillation. Her husband, daughter, and son-in-law were at home when the storm happened, and they were afraid that they would lose her. At the time of the interview she had experienced one additional ICD storm. She says the ICD storm experience has made her take better care of herself, especially with regard to getting more rest. She states that she worries about future shocks but prays they do not happen. Her faith in God has helped her recover, and she says she does not take life for granted.

*Case #5*

A 47-year-old white man with a history of cardiac arrest was walking to his mailbox 5 months after implant when his device shocked him. He touched the metal mailbox and felt like the shock was amplified by the contact with metal. It "felt like a baseball team was hitting [him] in the chest with their bats," and he says he started crying. No one else was present. He dropped his mail and fell to the ground from the impact of the next shock, sustaining a fractured hip from the fall. He received 22 shocks during this storm and states that he would not choose to receive an ICD again. He has not experienced anything similar to the pain of the storm other than the nearly monthly isolated shocks, which produce the same pain response as the storm. He rates the pain of his shocks as a 9.5 on a scale of 0 to 10. He thinks the storm has made him fearful of shocks and he walks very "lightly" with his walker to avoid triggering a shock. He perceives his wife and family as being supportive and helpful. He states that his family was upset that he had to be hospitalized for the broken hip.

*Case #6*

A 63-year-old white man with a history of coronary artery disease was working in his yard less than 1 month after implant when he experienced an ICD storm that involved 32 shocks. He says it "scared [him] to death" and "hurt worse than anything." He rated the pain score as a 10 on a scale of 0 to 10 and further described it "like a bomb going off inside me... and [he] saw blue lights like lightning with each shock." He says he "gets cold chills thinking about it" and compares it to the pain he experienced from an accidental gunshot wound to his chest. He had no warning signs or symptoms, and he was later told that atrial fibrillation was the cause of the ICD storm. His cardiologist provided a magnet to take home after the storm and instructed him in how to use it to stop the defibrillator. This instruction helped psychologically to give the patient a sense of control, but he has not used it. He has had several isolated shocks and another 12-shock storm experience since the original storm episode. The patient feels that the experience has the same level of intensity each time. He worries about the pain, which

has made him afraid to do many activities. He returned to work, which he feels has taken his mind off his fears and helped reduce financial worries. His family was "scared to death" and wanted to help but did not know what to do. Knowing that the ICD was adjusted after the storm helped him the most in terms of coping with the fear of future shocks.

## Comparison of patients with low (4 or fewer) and high (more than 4) numbers of storm shocks

In the Canadian Implantable Defibrillator study, quality of life was negatively affected only in subjects who received more than four shocks [22]. Pain perception and fear of future pain seemed to be the main characteristics that differed between these subsets of storm patients. All patients interviewed perceived subsequent shocks in the same manner as the initial storm shock experience. For example, if the first experience was not perceived as painful, then subsequent shocks were not described as painful. Likewise, most participants reported feeling afraid to exert themselves after a storm. Two particular phrases were used—"walking on eggshells" and "walking lightly"—to describe the response to fear of retriggering a shock. Helpful strategies to cope with the experience included returning to work and usual activities, relying on support of family and friends, and relying on faith in God. All participants say their families were concerned and supportive and that they had good relationships with nurses and doctors who treated them after the storm. Some patients said that their family members wanted to help but did not know what to do. Sensory descriptions of the storm experience varied greatly, with high shock patients reporting pain at 9.5 and 10 on a scale of 0 to 10 and low storm participants not reporting significant pain during the episodes. These distinctly different responses may suggest a dose-response effect with regard to sensory perception and storm.

## Immediate post-storm care

Upon initial encounter with a patient post ICD storm, it is important to assess a patient for any injuries that may have occurred during the storm event. Injuries are more likely in patients who are unsteady on their feet before the storm. Although physical injury takes precedence over dealing with the psychological aftermath of the storm, it is important to assess a patient's emotional state and provide initial reassurance. Evaluation of compliance with medications and prompt measurement of serum electrolytes also is critical.

Once a patient is stabilized, the primary nursing concerns are the patient's pain, fear, and possible lack of information. Pain is most often described by patients as moderate to severe and like a blow to the body or a spasm that causes the entire body to move [23,24]. Post-shock assessment includes obtaining a detailed history of the event, reviewing information retrieved from the device, and discussing psychological concerns and perceptions with the patient and family members. As with physical injury, emotional issues must be addressed appropriately to help the patient and family understand how stress may be a cause and a consequence of ICD shocks. Important areas of post-shock assessment are listed in Box 1.

Medical care after storm consists of a physical examination and appropriate treatment based on findings and analysis of the results of device interrogation. Patients with monomorphic ventricular arrhythmias may benefit from catheter ablation, a procedure that identifies and destroys arrhythmogenic cells. Marrouche et al [25] tested this technique on 29 patients who had storm caused by ventricular fibrillation and found that the borders of ischemic areas were appropriate targets for ablation. With more research, this type of technique may help to prevent recurrent storm. For patients with lead fracture, replacement and ICD revision are indicated.

## Device programming

A working knowledge of typical ICD programming is helpful when talking to a person who has experienced storm. Patients can be taught to understand the basics of their ICD settings, and it is reassuring for them to know that a device often can be reprogrammed to prevent further episodes of storm. This reassurance may be particularly helpful in the setting of inappropriate shocks from atrial fibrillation or sinus tachycardia. When appropriate shocks are delivered, several interventions are used to reduce future shocks, including activating or reprogramming the anti-tachycardia pacing scheme, starting or adjusting dosages of anti-arrhythmic drugs, correcting electrolyte depletion, and performing catheter ablation if the recorded arrhythmia is unifocal and accessible [26].

## Patient education

Patient education is an important strategy for facilitating recovery after storm. Because episodes may occur long after implant and initial patient teaching, a brief assessment of patient and family knowledge levels identifies educational needs and approaches. Problem-solving and information-gathering skills should be encouraged along with development of an "action plan" for dealing with future shocks. Misperceptions about causes of shocks and fear of potential future episodes must be addressed along with concerns about reduced battery life after storm. Battery life is affected by use, but most batteries last 5 years. Routine ICD checks ensure adequate time for battery replacement in the event of depletion. Phantom shocks also may occur, and patients should be encouraged to have their ICD checked if they are unsure if a shock was real or not. Family members often have unexpressed concerns and are emotionally affected by the ICD and surrounding circumstances [27]. They should have the opportunity to discuss issues with the caregiver in a private setting to facilitate full disclosure of concerns.

Careful listening and focusing on expressed concerns help target areas for short- and long-term education. Required nursing skills are psychological in nature and are similar to those used for patients with posttraumatic stress symptoms or other sudden,

---

**Box 1. Immediate post-storm assessment**

Assess for injury

Inquire about any missed doses of medications

Look for causes of electrolyte depletion: not taking prescribed potassium or magnesium supplements, diarrhea, anorexia

Ask patient how he or she was feeling just before the storm

Ask what activity the patient was doing when the storm occurred; assess for sources of electromagnetic interference

What does the patient think caused the storm?

Ask the patient if he or she ever had an experience like ICD storm before; look for similar past experiences that may add to the trauma of current experience

frightening experiences. Because ICD shocks are often life-saving, however, the opportunity for reducing emotional distress through timely education and therapeutic counseling should be greater than in traumatic situations, in which the stressor has no intrinsic benefit. Patients who have had storm may be given a magnet and instructions on how to deactivate the defibrillator in the event of reoccurring storm. This education provides an additional tool to help regain a sense of control over the unexpected event of storm, but some patients may fear that turning off the device will produce a worse outcome than storm, so counseling and step-by-step instructions are helpful. Rarely, storm may precipitate panic disorder, which is treatable with cognitive behavioral therapy [28,29]. Referral to a clinical psychologist or counselor for cognitive therapy has been shown to be effective in helping patients return to normal activity after storm [20,29].

## Patient counseling

Quality of life is reported to be worse in patients with ICDs who receive a shock [30]; however, only 5% of patients who were shocked say that they would rather not have the ICD after being shocked [23]. Responses to questions about storm may vary depending on when the ICD storm occurred. Important variables to consider when talking to people who have experienced ICD storm are the duration of time since storm and the number of shocks experienced. Initially, some patients may have negative feelings about the device but later may report satisfaction with the ICD, realizing its positive effects and benefits.

The psychological side effects of storm can lead to physical and emotional symptoms that may present like posttraumatic stress or panic disorder, depending on how many shocks were received and how the person perceived the experience. In a study by Dunbar et al [24], 87% of participants who received shocks reported feeling nervous afterwards, and participants who received multiple shocks had greater concerns than persons who received isolated shocks. Social embarrassment and lack of control over the situation should be explored and discussed with patients who have experienced storm to normalize the experience. Talking to other patients who have experienced storm may be beneficial.

Assessing for irrational associations between shocks and activities or thoughts is important in preventing unnecessary reductions in activity among patients who have had storm. Patients may associate shock therapy with a decline in health and thereby

create a reinforced sense of illness [20]. Clarification from practitioners regarding a patient's change in physical condition as it relates to the storm should be provided for patients and family members after appropriate examination and testing. In some cases in which the recipient of ICD or biventricular ICD has a terminal illness, deactivation of the ICD may be indicated as a solution for emotional issues after electrical storm if quality of life is demonstrably decreased [31,32]. As part of a permanent or upon-admission living will, patients also may want to consider including specific advance directives concerning situations in which they wish their device to be deactivated. Details of patient education and counseling are listed in Box 2.

---

**Box 2. Important points for implantable cardioverter defibrillator storm patient education and counseling**

- Assess patient and family member knowledge about ICD purpose and self-care
- Clarify cause of ICD storm; provide information regarding prevention, including medication adherence, having serum electrolytes checked as indicated, eating a healthy diet, and taking prescribed supplements to prevent electrolyte depletion
- Discuss reprogramming of device and other strategies that were performed to prevent future shocks
- If appropriate, offer patient a magnet and instructions on how to deactivate the ICD for recurrent storm
- Assess patient and family members' perception of patient's health status and changes; encourage optimal physical and social functioning
- Discuss phantom shocks and encourage patients to have device checked if unsure about a shock
- Clarify activity recommendations
- Talk to family members separately from patients to allow full disclosure of concerns; encourage family planning for patient's discharge and return to activities

## Summary

ICDs and biventricular ICDs are the mainstay of treatment for life-threatening ventricular arrhythmia and will become even more common in the near future. Device complexity increases with each new model, which allows more programming options and potential therapeutic benefit for patients but also increases the challenge for clinicians to stay current on technologic improvements and patient responses. ICD storm occurs infrequently; however, it warrants timely medical intervention, psychological debriefing, and patient and family education to prevent long-term emotional and subsequent physical consequences. Patient responses to storm vary greatly and may be dose dependent, particularly regarding the pain response. Injury can occur as a result of storm, which further complicates the clinical picture and possibly the emotional response to perceived ICD benefit. Clinicians have a responsibility to educate patients carefully about the shock experience to make them aware that shocks are painful but brief and let them know that device reprogramming and anti-arrhythmic therapy may be needed at some point. The opportunity to talk with other recipients of ICDs may increase support and access to information. Patients should be encouraged to learn as much as possible about the functions of the ICD, how to live a healthy life, and maintain maximum physical and social functioning with the implanted device.

## References

[1] Moss AJ, Zareba W, Hall WJ, et al. The multicenter automatic defibrillator implantation trial II investigators: prophylactic implantation of a defibrillator in patients with myocardial infarction and reduced ejection fraction. N Engl J Med 2002;346:877–83.

[2] Essebag V, Eisenberg MJ. Expanding indications for defibrillators after myocardial infarction: risk stratification and cost effectiveness. Card Electrophysiol Rev 2003;7(1):43–8.

[3] Seidl K, Senges J. Worldwide utilization of implantable cardioverter/defibrillators now and in the future. Card Electrophysiol Rev 2003;7(1):5–13.

[4] Klein HAA, Reek S, Geller C. New primary prevention trials of sudden cardiac death in patients with left ventricular dysfunction: SCD-HEFT and MADIT-II. Am J Cardiol 1999;83(91):91D–7D.

[5] Medtronic. SCD-Heft Fact Sheet. Available at: http://www.medtronic.com/downloadablefiles/SCD-HeFT%20-%20Fact%20Sheet.pdf 2004. Accessed July 16, 2004.

[6] DiMarco JP. Medical progress: implantable cardioverter-defibrillators. N Engl J Med 2003;349(19):1836–47.

[7] Saxon LA, Ellenbogen KA. Resynchronization therapy for the treatment of heart failure. Circulation 2003; 108(9):1044–8.

[8] Credner SC, Klingenheben T, Mauss O, et al. Electrical storm in patients with transvenous implantable cardioverter-defibrillators: incidence, management and prognostic implications. J Am Coll Cardiol 1998;32(7): 1909–15.

[9] Korte T, Jung W, Ostermann G, et al. Hospital readmission in patients with modern implantable cardioverter/defibrillators [abstract]. Pacing Clin Electrophysiol 1997;20:1207.

[10] Lampert R, McPherson CA, Clancy JF, et al. Gender differences in ventricular arrhythmia recurrence in patients with coronary artery disease and implantable cardioverter-defibrillators. J Am Coll Cardiol 2004;43(12):2293–9.

[11] Exner D, Pinski S, Wyse D, et al. Electrical storm presages nonsudden death: the antiarrhythmics versus implantable defibrillators (AVID) trial. Circulation 2001;103(16):2066–71.

[12] Kadish A, Dyer A, Daubert JP, et al. Prophylactic defibrillator implantation in patients with nonischemic dilated cardiomyopathy. N Engl J Med 2004;350(21): 2151–8.

[13] Bristow MR, Saxon LA, Boehmer J, et al. Cardiac-resynchronization therapy with or without an implantable defibrillator in advanced chronic heart failure. N Engl J Med 2004;350(21):2140–50.

[14] Kouakam C, Kacet S, Hazard JR, et al. Performance of a dual-chamber implantable defibrillator algorithm for discrimination of ventricular from supraventricular tachycardia. Europace 2004;6(1):32–42.

[15] Whang W, Mittleman MA, Rich DQ, et al. Heart failure and the risk of shocks in patients with implantable cardioverter defibrillators: results from the triggers of ventricular arrhythmias (TOVA) study. Circulation 2004;109(11):1386–91.

[16] Swerdlow CD, Schsls W, Dijkman B, et al. Detection of atrial fibrillation and flutter by a dual-chamber implantable cardioverter-defibrillator. Circulation 2000; 101(8):878–85.

[17] Rinaldi Sr CA, Baszko A, Bostock J, et al. A 17 year experience of inappropriate shock therapy in patients with implantable cardioverter-defibrillators: are we getting any better? Heart 2004;90:330–1.

[18] Bocciardo MAM, Gaita F, Trappe HJ, et al. Efficacy of biventricular sensing and treatment of ventricular tachycardia. Pacing Clin Electrophysiol 2000;23 1989–91.

[19] Schron EB, Exner DV, Yao Q, et al. Quality of life in the antiarrhythmics versus implantable defibrillators trial: impact of therapy and influence of adverse symptoms and defibrillator shocks. Circulation 2002; 105(5):589–94.

[20] Sears Jr SE, Conti JB. Understanding implantable cardioverter defibrillator shocks and storms: medical and psychosocial considerations for research and clinical care. Clin Cardiol 2003;26(3):107–11.

[21] Dunbar SB, O'Brien MC, Kimble L, et al. Implantable cardioverter defibrillator activity and psychological outcomes. Heart Rhythm 2004;1(1 Suppl):s252–3.

[22] Irvine JDP, Baker B, O'Brien BJ, et al. Quality of life in the Canadian implantable defibrillator study (CIDS). Am Heart J 2002;144:282–9.

[23] Ahmad M, Bloomstein L, Roelke M, et al. Patients' attitudes toward implanted defibrillator shocks. Pacing Clin Electrophysiol 2000;23(6):934–8.

[24] Dunbar SB, Warner CD, Purcell JA. Internal cardioverter defibrillator device discharge: experiences of patients and family members. Heart Lung 1993;22:494–501.

[25] Marrouche NF, Verma A, Wazni O, et al. Mode of initiation and ablation of ventricular fibrillation storms in patients with ischemic cardiomyopathy. J Am Coll Cardiol 2004;43(9):1715–20.

[26] Miller JM, Hsia HH. Management of the patient with frequent discharges from implantable cardioverter defibrillator devices. J Cardiovasc Electrophysiol 1996;7:278–85.

[27] Marx A, Bollman A, Dunbar S, et al. Psychological reactions among family members of patients with implantable defibrillators. Int J Psychiatry Med 2001;31(4):375–87.

[28] Neu P, Godemann F. First onset of panic disorder and agoraphobia induced by a series of inappropriate shocks of an implanted cardioverter/defibrillator. Nervenarzt 2003;74(3):266–8.

[29] Sears Jr SF, Rauch S, Handberg E, et al. Fear of exertion following ICD storm: considering ICD shock and learning history. J Cardiopulm Rehabil 2001;21(1):47–9.

[30] McCready MJ, Exner DV. Quality of life and psychological impact of implantable cardioverter defibrillators: focus on randomized controlled trial data. Card Electrophysiol Rev 2003;7(1):63–70.

[31] DiMarco JP. Implantable cardioverter-defibrillators and complications [correspondence]. N Engl J Med 2004;350(7):734–5.

[32] Sinclair CT. Implantable cardioverter-defibrillators and complications [correspondence]. N Engl J Med 2004;350(7):734–5.

ELSEVIER
SAUNDERS

Crit Care Nurs Clin N Am 17 (2005) 17–22

CRITICAL CARE
NURSING CLINICS
OF NORTH AMERICA

# Pediatric Post-resuscitation Care

Shirley W. Cantrell, PhD, RN*, Karen S. Ward, PhD, RN

*School of Nursing, Middle Tennessee State University, Box 81, Murfreesboro, TN 37132, USA*

Few recent articles address the issue of caring for children after cardiopulmonary resuscitation (CPR). One explanation might be the low incidence of cardiac arrest (12.7 per 100,000) in children under 18 years of age [1]. Another possible reason is that the outcome of pediatric CPR can be poor [2,3], which theoretically leaves care after CPR unnecessary. Reliable reporting mechanisms and national information archives have been inconsistent until recently, when the National Register of Cardiopulmonary Resuscitation, sponsored by the American Heart Association, was established [3,4].

As with any "low incidence" situation, the desirability of high-quality and appropriate care is implicit, regardless of the number of individuals it affects. The goal is not only successful resuscitation. Children and their families need holistic care that meets all of their needs after a life-altering experience. Families need assistance in dealing with the situation if the resuscitation was unsuccessful.

Key issues involved with post-resuscitation care include (1) the outcome of CPR, (2) immediate post-resuscitation needs, (3) emotional outcomes for the child, and (4) the stress and grief experienced by the family. Nurses are involved intimately in all of these areas. Many independent nursing actions can contribute significantly to positive outcomes for the children and their families.

## Outcome of pediatric cardiopulmonary resuscitation

Zaritsky [2] stated that in most cases, pediatric patients with cardiac arrest either die or survive with significant neurologic damage. Many children experience respiratory depression and arrest as the initial insult. In pediatric patients, cardiac arrest is often secondary to hypoxemia. The severity and duration of hypoxemia sufficient to stop the heart also have severe effects on the cerebral cortex [5]. In 1983, Eisenberg et al [1] found that successful pediatric resuscitation occurred only 7% of the time. There was no information on the condition of the children after resuscitation.

In 1986, Gillis et al [5] investigated long-term survival after cardiac arrest. The study followed the children through initial resuscitation, hospital stay, and 6 months later. The findings of this study showed that only 9% of children survived 6 months after cardiac arrest. This is in contrast to another study conducted during the same year [6], which noted that only 2% to 20% of children survived cardiac arrest, and most of the survivors suffered neurologic impairment.

Additional studies indicated that survival rates were as low as zero to 17%, even with aggressive resuscitation. Morris and Nadkami [7] found that the initial return of spontaneous circulation after cardiac arrest was 5% to 64%; of the survivors, 20% to 83% had significant neurologic impairment. With progressive deterioration in cardiopulmonary function leading to cardiac arrest in children, the degree of ischemia and acidosis is severe.

Some recent studies have suggested a more optimistic outcome [3,4]. As more reliable report-

* Corresponding author.
*E-mail address:* swcantre@mtsu.edu (S.W. Cantrell).

ing mechanisms are developed, perhaps additional research can lead to ways for continuing an increased success rate. Nurses in the hospital can assist in improved data collection and reporting. Persons in the community also can contribute by conducting good case follow-up and reporting out-of-hospital incidents.

## Immediate post-resuscitation care

Immediate post-resuscitation care includes measures to optimize cardiac output and cerebral perfusion, match oxygen and substrate delivery to meet metabolic needs, minimize reperfusion injury, and support cellular recovery. Injured cells can hibernate, die, partially recover, or fully recover. The rehabilitation phase after cardiac arrest focuses on salvaging injured cells, recruiting hibernating cells, and reengineering partially recovered cells [7,8].

There has been controversy over the use of sodium bicarbonate to correct acidosis. When sodium bicarbonate is used to neutralize acidosis, the end products are water and carbon dioxide. Because respirations are compromised during CPR, the carbon dioxide builds up and causes further acidosis that adversely affects the neurologic outcome [8,9]. Outwater et al [6] noted that complications from the use of sodium bicarbonate included hypernatremia, hyperosmolality, hypercarbia, cerebrospinal fluid acidosis, and inhibition of oxygen release into tissues. Close assessment for signs of these complications should be part of the plan of care if sodium bicarbonate is used during resuscitation.

Hyperventilation has been used to reduce the carbon dioxide levels after resuscitation; however, it may lead to increased cerebral vasoconstriction, ischemia, and a worsening condition [10]. The sudden increase in the partial pressure of oxygen that often occurs after resuscitation may contribute to reperfusion injury by creating excessive free radicals. Animal studies are being conducted to identify the benefit of administering antioxidants after resuscitation to decrease free radicals [7]. A second way to decrease free radicals is to resuscitate with room air. Studies have been conducted in delivery room resuscitation of newborns with room air and with oxygen. No difference in outcomes was noted [7].

Temperature management is important after resuscitation; even mild hyperthermia is associated with a poor outcome [7]. To improve the outcome, a mild hypothermia may be induced. Two other methods to combat the dangers of hyperthermia are the administration of antipyretic medications according to a set schedule and the use of external cooling devices [4,7]. Keeping a constant watch on the child's temperature is an important nursing activity.

Cell damage from cerebral anoxia initiates the inflammatory process, which causes cerebral edema. Frequent assessment for signs of increased intercranial pressure should be included in the nursing plan of care [11]. Neurologic problems that might result include weakness in the extremities, loss of memory, confusion, restlessness, and incomprehensible speech. Monitoring of these signs and symptoms is vital for an optimal outcome.

During post-resuscitative care, communication with the patient is critical, especially if a ventilator is required for respiratory management. Careful age-appropriate explanations of all procedures and information about the machines help calm the child. Explaining to children why they cannot talk or move around much with an endotracheal tube inserted helps alleviate anxiety, even if it does not make them happy. Helping them understand that the situation is temporary and that letting the machine breathe for them until they are strong enough to breathe on their own is also beneficial. It is important to develop other methods of communication, such as pointing at pictures for children who cannot yet read and write. Providing a slate for written communication for children who can write is a common nursing intervention. Extensive communication with and education of the family also is an integral part of caring for a child with a ventilator after cardiac arrest.

Assessment of renal function is also desirable. The child should be on strict intake and output. Excessive fluid may exacerbate the cerebral edema and create additional stress on the heart. The decreased or nonexistent blood flow to the kidneys during CPR also could cause acute renal failure. Observing for appropriate intake and output balance is essential in caring for a child after resuscitation.

Autoregulation of cerebral blood flow is impaired after cardiac arrest, which may lead to difficulty maintaining cerebral perfusion or inability to protect the brain from acute hypertension [7]. Blood pressure variability should be minimized after resuscitation. Animal studies have demonstrated improved neurologic outcomes with brief hypertension after CPR [7].

Administration of insulin and glucose ensures adequate energy for brain function. These substances have been shown to improve neurologic outcome. Judicious oversight of blood glucose levels is necessary to prevent hyper- or hypoglycemia [4].

The endothelial damage to blood vessels that occurs during CPR causes the release of von Willebrand factor and increases tissue thromboplastin. The resulting platelet aggregation causes microvascular thrombi, which leads to further ischemia of tissue throughout the body and results in multiorgan dysfunction. This occurrence may indicate a future role of thrombolytic agents during post-resuscitation care. Monitoring for signs of ischemic tissue or organ problems is crucial.

## Emotional outcome for the child after cardiac arrest

In addition to the potential physical problems that critically ill children may face, there are numerous difficult philosophical, psychological, and religious challenges. These challenges must be met with openness and candor. Children and their families must feel free to confront these problems as readily as they deal with the physical ones [12].

Children under stress from illness may find it difficult to see themselves as independent from the family. Progressive independence is natural as children advance through developmental states, and severe illness is a threat to that progression [13]. On the other hand, some children may experience feelings of isolation and distance because of their departure from the normal routine that the family had before the manifestation of illness. Encouraging children to express feelings of frustration regarding any effects of their situation is useful.

For young children, being separated from the family represents a frightening loss of self. Older children may feel helpless, uncertain of the disease and treatment outcomes, and unsure of the impact their illness might have on the balance in the family system. They may be well aware of neurologic deficits and may experience conflict at not being able to fulfill their role in the family [13].

Emotional distress and suffering in ill children also may stem from an altered body self-concept. It is a frightening experience when their body is disfigured, examined, or changed in any way. This stress and suffering may go unnoticed unless specific information is elicited. A child's withdrawal, sadness, anger, loneliness, and frustration can be mistakenly attributed to the fear of the hospital setting rather than the perceived changed relationships with others and self [12,13]. Difficulty in sleeping, irritability, not eating, and withdrawal can be physical manifestations of this distress and suffering.

Another facet of emotional care may arise if a child has a near-death experience during resuscitation. Several researchers have documented that near death experiences occur in children of all ages

---

**Box 1. Common elements of near death experience in children**

Experiencing an out-of-body feeling
Hearing buzzing or rushing water
Entering into a void or tunnel
Seeing or entering into bright spiritual light
Encountering a border or limit
Perceiving return to the body as a conscious choice or forced event [15]

---

[14–19]. Common elements have been found to exist regarding near-death experiences in children (Box 1). Children who report these spiritual visions are often stigmatized as being irrational and absurd; however, these experiences are vividly real to the children. Many adults and health care personnel are uncomfortable talking to children about death and visions. Children may be afraid to talk about their experiences for fear of being labeled as crazy. It is important to allow children to relate what they have perceived. If they are not allowed to talk freely, they withdraw and wonder about this experience in silence [20].

Atwater [14] has described a "brain shift" that often occurs after a near-death experience. Children can exhibit no fear of death and a love of inspiring music and solitude. There is also an increased sensitivity to light, sound, foods, and drinks. This reaction could interfere with activities of daily living. Some children have developed prolific psychic abilities [14]. Many have a transformation in value systems and increased concern for others [17].

Near-death experiences can create a wide variety of difficult emotional issues for the children who have them and for their parents. It is important that health care professionals do not trivialize or dismiss them as fantasies or hallucinations. Children must be listened to and validated by health care professionals. Families need assistance in understanding what their child has gone through and in discovering ways to talk together about it. If families can develop such effective communication skills, future problems, such as posttraumatic stress disorder and depression, hopefully can be averted [12].

The attained language development of the child may affect the likelihood of capturing complete and accurate descriptions of near-death experiences [19]. One method of allowing a young child to express this experience is through play and drawing. These are good media for children to communicate internal feelings that they may have difficulty putting into words [13]. Drawing also can work for older children, but they also have the ability to write about their thoughts and feelings in a journal. The contents of the journal can be shared or not as the child wishes, because the writing itself can be therapeutic. It is important for nurses to develop interventions that support children and their families as they work through these experiences.

## Family stress and grief

Families are also under stress and bear the responsibility of making decisions for their ill child. Ethical decision making involves issues that are complex and profound dealing with emotionally charged questions [21,22]. Parents also experience anticipatory grief when there is neurologic damage that occurs with so many children who survive resuscitation. This damage may necessitate reorganization of lifestyle for the family. Parents may experience an altered relationship with their child that results from the child's internal changes after a resuscitation event. If neurologic damage occurs, parents' hopes and dreams for their child's future may need to be altered [23].

Another controversial issue that may impact the family is family presence during resuscitation. Most family members want to be present during resuscitation of their child [10,24]. The benefits to the family being present during resuscitation include knowing everything is being done for their child and feeling that they are supporting and helping the child with their presence. It also reduces their anxiety and fear and allows them to maintain a connectedness with their child. If the child does not survive, it gives them some closure and facilitates their grieving [25].

Mason [26] states that not enough is known about the psychological impact that being present during resuscitation would have on the family to make policy decisions at this time. Increasing numbers of institutions are allowing family to be present, however, because of support of professional organizations, attention of the media, and research on the topic [27]. A lot rests on the attitudes of staff members regarding the issue and their willingness to have the family in the room. Nurses must be comfortable with their own role to provide the kind of support family members need if they are going to be prepared to witness their child's resuscitation. Some form of education if the possibility of an arrest exists or postevent debriefing contributes to the value

of the experience of any family member who might remain in the room [24].

Because a large percentage of pediatric cardiac arrests result in the death of the child, caring for the grieving family becomes part of post-resuscitation care. When a child dies, it violates one of the basic laws of nature: that parents should precede their children in death [22]. Several characteristics of a child's death influence the parents' grief and are important to note (Box 2). Grieving for a child affects the marital relationship. Women are allowed to grieve more openly than men. Societies send the message to men that they must be strong and take care of their spouse, which can lead to dysfunctional grieving and friction in the family.

Siblings also grieve the dead child. The expressions of grief vary with age, experience with prior losses, relationship with their sibling, individual personality, perceptions surrounding the loss, and the meaning the loss has for them. The most powerful influence, however, is the parents' response to the loss [22]. Nurses must address these issues with the family after the death of a child.

One of the first tasks of mourners is accepting the loss. Seeing and holding their child after death helps parents conceptually confirm the child's death. Brown and Bocock [10] found that 88% of the parents in their study felt that viewing their child's body was helpful in their grieving. Ninety-three percent wanted a memento, hand- or footprint, lock of hair, or photo; 65% thought that "follow-up" would be helpful.

One such follow-up is described in the literature as a grief conferment. This meeting takes place 4 to 6 weeks after the child has died. The family decides who they want to attend the conference—usually physicians and nurses who cared for their child. The

---

**Box 2. Characteristics of a child's death that influence parents' grief**

- The situation surrounding the death
- The timeliness of the death
- The parents' perception of the preventability of the death
- Whether the death was sudden, unexpected, or anticipated
- The length of illness before death
- The amount of parental anticipatory grief
- The degree of involvement with the child [23]

conference gives the health care team the opportunity to give the family the autopsy report if there is one and a chance to assess how the family is doing. It gives the family the opportunity to ask questions they were unable to ask at the time that their child died [22].

Brown and Sefansky [28] describe the development of a bereavement committee, whose mission is to develop the expertise needed to provide a high quality of bereavement care to the child and the family. The committee, which is multidisciplinary and includes nurses, social workers, chaplains, and physicians, designed a bereavement packet to be given to the family by the nurse or social worker, who spends time with the family immediately after the child's death. The packet contains in writing much of what the nurse or social worker tells the family about grief and provides books, poems, and phone numbers for support groups. They also have designed a follow-up program to remain in contact with the family through cards and calls throughout the year after the child's death. The goals of the bereavement committee are to offer support, education, and resources to the staff, help the families through the immediate crisis of the child's death, and offer ongoing support and resources to the family for a year after the child's death [28].

## Summary

Despite the lack of current literature, it is apparent that properly caring for children after a resuscitation event can contribute significantly to a positive outcome. Children and their families need to receive expert physical and emotional treatment for optimal results. Nurses are the main providers of such care. Further inquiry and research into this area is sorely needed. As better records of the actual incidence of pediatric cardiac arrest occurrences are kept and made available, better ways of dealing with the event itself and postevent care can be developed. Subsequent use of such findings allows nurses to provide the best care possible for this population.

## References

[1] Eisenberg M, Bergner L, Hallstrom A. Epidemiology of cardiac arrest in children. Ann Emerg Med 1983; 12(11):272–4.

[2] Zaritsky A. Pediatric resuscitation pharmacology. Ann Emerg Med 1993;22(2 Pt 2):445–55.

[3] National Registry of CardioPulmonary Resuscitation.

About the National Registry of CardioPulmonary Resuscitation. Available at: http://www.nrcpr.org. Accessed August 10, 2004.

[4] Chadwick VL, Arrowsmith JE. Recent advances in pediatric resuscitation. Pediatr Anesthesia 2004;14: 417–20.

[5] Gillis J, Dickson D, Rieder M, et al. Results of in-patient pediatric resuscitation. Crit Care Med 1986; 14(5):469–71.

[6] Outwater KM, Ludwig S, Peterson MB. Pediatric resuscitation. J Emerg Nurs 1989;15(6):466–74.

[7] Morris MC, Nadkami VM. Pediatric cardiopulmonary-cerebral resuscitation: an overview and future directions. Crit Care Clin 2003;19(3):537–64.

[8] Ushay HM, Notterman DA. Pharmacology of pediatric resuscitation. Pediatr Clin North Am 1997;44(1): 207–33.

[9] Zaritsky A. Selected concepts and controversies in pediatric cardiopulmonary resuscitation. Crit Care Clin 1988;4(4):735–54.

[10] Brown K, Bocock J. Update in pediatric resuscitation. Emerg Med Clin North Am 2002;20(1):1–26.

[11] Vaughan R. Intensive care following cardiac arrest. Nurs Times 1982;78(44):1843–5.

[12] McInyk BM, Small L, Carno MA. The effectiveness of parent-focused interventions in improving coping/mental health outcomes of critically ill children and their parents: an evidence base to guide clinical practice. Pediatr Nurs 2004;30(2):143–8.

[13] Sparta SN. Suffering by children: some observations of brave children and their families at a children's hospital. Loss, Grief & Care 1988;2(3/4):81–93.

[14] Atwater PMH. Children and the near-death phenomenon: another viewpoint. Journal of Near-Death Studies 1996;15(1):5–16.

[15] Morse MI. Near death experiences and death-related visions in children: implications for the children. Curr Probl Pediatr 1994;24(2):55–83.

[16] Serdahely WJ. Loving help from the other side: a mosaic of some near-death, and near-death-like, experiences. Journal of Near-Death Studies 1992; 10(3):171–82.

[17] McEvoy MD. The near-death experience: implications for nursing education. Loss Grief Care 1990;4(1/2): 51–5.

[18] Serdahely WJ. Pediatric near-death experiences. Journal of Near-Death Studies 1990;9(1):33–9.

[19] Bush NE. The near-death experience in children: shades of the prison-house reopening. Anabiosis 1983; 3(2):177–93.

[20] Raimbault G. Children talk about death. Acta Paediatr Scand 1981;70(2):179–82.

[21] Golub ZD. Loss of the "perfect" child and ethical decision making: Miguel's story. Loss Grief Care 1988; 2(3/4):27–32.

[22] Wheeler SR, Pike MM. Families' responses to the loss of a child. In: Fawcett CS, editor. Family psychiatric nursing. Chicago: Mosby; 1993. p. 140–61.

[23] Linder CM, Suddaby EC, Mowery BD. Parental pres-

ence during resuscitation: help or hindrance? Pediatr
Nurs 2004;30(2):126–7, 148.

[24] Curtis JR, Engelberg RA, Wenrich MD, et al. Studying
communication about end-of-life care during the
ICU family conference: development of a framework.
J Crit Care 2002;17(3):147–80.

[25] Eichhorn DJ, Meyers TA, Guzzetta CE, et al. Family
presence during invasive procedures and resuscitation:
hearing the voice of the patient. Am J Nurs 2001;
101(5):48–55.

[26] Mason DJ. Family presence: evidence versus tradition.
Am J Crit Care 2003;12(3):190–2.

[27] MacLean SL, Guzzetta E, White C, et al. Family
presence during cardiopulmonary resuscitation and
invasive procedures: practices of critical care and
emergency nurses. Am J Crit Care 2003;12(3):246–57.

[28] Brown PS, Sefansky S. Enhancing bereavement care
in the pediatric ICU. Crit Care Nurs 1995;15(5):62–4.

ELSEVIER
SAUNDERS

Crit Care Nurs Clin N Am 17 (2005) 23–32

CRITICAL CARE
NURSING CLINICS
OF NORTH AMERICA

# Family Presence During Cardiopulmonary Resuscitation

Angela P. Clark, PhD, RN, CNS, FAAN, FAHA[a,*],
Michael D. Aldridge, MSN, RN, CCRN[b],
Cathie E. Guzzetta, PhD, RN, HNC, FAAN[c],
Patty Nyquist- Heise, RN, BSN, CCRN[d], Reverend Mike Norris[d],
Patti Loper, RN, BA, CHRN[d], Theresa A. Meyers, MS, BSN, RN, CEN[d],
Wayne Voelmeck, MSN, RN[a]

[a]University of Texas at Austin School of Nursing, 1700 Red River, Austin, TX 78701, USA
[b]Children's Hospital of Austin, 1400 North I.H.35, Austin, TX 78701, USA
[c]Children's Medical Center of Dallas, 1935 Motor Street, Dallas, TX 75235, USA
[d]Memorial Hospital, 1400 East Boulder Street, Colorado Springs, CO 80909, USA

Providing family-centered care is not always a simple endeavor [1], and creating this culture usually requires time and patience. One of the most distinctive forms of family support has emerged in various acute care settings in the United States, initially beginning in the emergency department and slowly diffusing to other areas, such as the intensive care unit (ICU). Allowing family members to remain at a patient's bedside during resuscitation is a relatively new concept [2] and is controversial in most institutions. Health care providers' attitudes and experiences with family presence (FP) have been the subject of several studies, primarily about nurses and physicians [2–22]. Compelling findings about the positive reactions of family members who experience FP also have been reported [2,23–33]. The emerging trends showing benefits to the family unit have astounded some health care providers who are opposed to it and have reassured others who instinctively embrace it. This article explores the state of the science about FP during resuscitation events and proposes some unique implementation strategies.

## Cardiopulmonary resuscitation outcomes as context for family presence

The outcomes of cardiopulmonary resuscitation (CPR) are an important part of the context in which FP must be evaluated. The words "grim" and "dismal" are often used to describe survival statistics after cardiopulmonary arrests, which are reported to be less than 17% for in-hospital arrests [34] and 1% to 20% for out-of-hospital arrests [35]. Researchers in a recent study reported that for patients in the hospital who suffer an unwitnessed cardiac arrest with initial rhythm that is not ventricular tachycardia or fibrillation and whose resuscitation lasts longer than 10 minutes, the survival rate is zero [36]. Although improved CPR outcomes from deployment of automated external defibrillators is encouraging, shortening the time to defibrillation remains to be the primary target for success [37].

The fascinating history of CPR itself may explain partially the reluctance of some health care providers to involve family members in viewing it or participating in it [38]. Developed and promoted in the 1960s, CPR was strictly for use only by physicians. Soon after Kouwenhoven et al [39] published their seminal article about cardiac massage, nonphysicians, including fire fighters, nurses, and the general public,

0899-5885/05/$ – see front matter © 2005 Elsevier Inc. All rights reserved.
doi:10.1016/j.ccell.2004.09.004

were intrigued with this simple technique that could reverse sudden deaths [38]. During that decade, controlling the teaching of lay people until physicians were comfortable with the technique spurred a debate [38].

Fortunately, non–health care providers continue to be slowly incorporated into the culture of resuscitation events and recognized for the parts they play. Current evidence about cardiopulmonary arrests suggests an even greater role for layperson responders than previously recognized. Two recent studies demonstrated improved outcomes based on the timely interventions initiated by volunteer citizens who performed CPR when they witnessed a cardiac arrest [40,41]. Other studies have shown that the odds of survival double when CPR is promptly administered by bystanders [42]. Some instances of FP have been described by family members as a logical and natural extension because of the CPR they did at home until the arrival of emergency medical services. Meyers et al [2] reported that in one third of the cases of FP during resuscitation, family members were with the patient during the onset, which occurred in an out-of-hospital setting, and assisted in summoning help and giving aid.

## What is family presence?

The most commonly used definition of FP is from the Emergency Nurses Association (ENA), which developed the original guidelines for emergency department nurses that were first published in 1995 and revised in 2001 [43,44]. These guidelines define FP as "the presence of family in the patient care area, in a location that affords visual or physical contact with the patient during invasive procedures or resuscitation events" [44]. These guidelines define family members as individuals who are relatives or significant others with whom the patient shares an established relationship [44].

Family member assessment and preparation must be part of the FP experience [44]. Not every family member wants the experience and must be supported in that choice. A landmark study of FP published in 2000 tested implementation of the ENA guidelines for FP and added criteria for family screening for study purposes, including the absence of combativeness, extreme emotional instability, and behaviors that suggested intoxication or altered mental status [2]. Suspected child abuse is another indication for not offering the family the opportunity for FP [45]. In the study by Meyers et al [2], 13% of family members who were assessed as suitable candidates for FP

declined the visitation option. Family members who participated in the study confirmed the power of FP, however. Researchers evaluated family member attitudes and beliefs 2 months after the FP event with telephone interviews, and 97% of the family members said they felt they had a right to be there and would do it again [2].

## History of family presence as an intervention

Where did this all begin? Although FP is a relatively new phenomenon to many critical care nurses and other health care providers, investigation of the origins of FP show that it is actually more than 20 years old. In 1982, pioneers working at W.A. Foote Memorial Hospital in Jackson, Michigan allowed family members to stay with their loved ones during CPR during two different encounters [8,22]. As a result of the positive feedback from persons who participated in the experience, leaders from the emergency department decided to study the phenomenon more closely. Using a clever idea for further analysis, they conducted a retrospective survey of family members of recently deceased patients to query their thoughts about whether they would have wanted to be present during CPR if given the chance. Members of 13 of the 18 families (72%) confirmed that they wished they had been present during the code [22]. Leaders proceeded to engage the staff in the possibility of FP and soon implemented an ongoing program of FP based on their findings.

A patient's family is an important social context, and caregivers must conceptualize the patient as existing within an integrated system of interdependent relationships [46]. Families are on their life journeys together regardless of the day-to-day operations of acute care hospitals. Kirchhoff et al [47] studied family members' experiences with death in the ICU and found a responsibility to protect and a strong desire to be with their loved one. Family members spoke of the importance of having a chance to say goodbye, and regrets lingered with them about missed opportunities. Merlevede et al [48] reported findings from a study of 74 relatives of 53 people with a sudden unexpected death, most of whom died at home, treated by emergency medical services. Some relatives who witnessed the event had left the room for fear of disturbing the interventions and afterward regretted not having given support to their loved one. New guidelines were added after the study to permit relatives who were willing to be present at the resuscitation at home to be allowed to attend.

## Case #1: a nurse's father

The following case study was written by an emergency department nurse as an exemplar about one of her many experiences with FP.

The emergency department was bursting at the seams with patients waiting to be seen. The acuity was high and the staff was stressed. The wait was long. A patient with a gunshot wound to the chest had just arrived in the trauma bay. We received a radio patch preparing us for an incoming patient with a cardiac arrest. The emergency medical services personnel stated that the patient had slumped over while playing bridge with friends at the Veterans Club. They had attempted three rounds of acute cardiac life support (ACLS) protocol without response. The family would arrive by car. Our team gathered in wait. On arrival we received a cyanotic, cold man. He was intubated, and CPR was in progress. The outcome looked grim as the team worked vigorously in an attempt to restore a pulse. We knew the family would be arriving soon. Most code situations are sudden and the family is in a state of shock. They are not prepared for loss of their loved one.

At our hospital, we believe that FP during resuscitation helps the family begin the grief process. We bring the family members into the room and, if possible, allow them close to the bed. A staff member assists with explanation of the procedures as they occur. It is hard for physicians and staff to tell a family that their loved one has died, especially if it is an unexpected event. Having them in the room during resuscitation seems to help prepare them for a bad outcome.

The call came that the wife had arrived. As we walked, I tried to prepare her for what she was about to visualize. They met in Germany and had been married for more than 50 years. As we entered the room, she saw staff still working to revive life in the body lying before her. Slowly I was able to move a chair close to the bed. She held his cold hand. She told the staff how he was such a good cook, and what a wonderful husband and father he had been. At first the team was tense, but as she shared her stories about her husband, the team was drawn to her. We felt the love that she and her husband had shared for each other.

As the resuscitation continued she looked over at me and said, "It's been too long, hasn't it?" I nodded in response. She then looked at the physician and told him, "It's okay, I know you've done all you can." The efforts were stopped, and the physician pronounced the patient dead. The machines were turned off; the room was quiet. She and I sat beside her husband and talked. She shared precious memories. That lifeless body became real to me. Soon her son arrived. She looked gently up at him and said. "Son, they did all they could. It just wasn't meant to be. I am so happy the last few minutes of his life were spent doing the thing he enjoyed most, playing cards with his friends."

We remained in the room for a while longer. The chaplain came for a short time to be with the family. We then walked to the parking lot. They hugged me and asked me to thank the staff for all their efforts. The next day, I received a call from the daughter, a military ICU nurse. She told me her mother shared how she was able to be with her husband during the resuscitation. She thanked me. As an intensive care nurse, the daughter stated that she also believed in FP. She felt it had made all the difference for her mother. After the funeral, I received a visit from the daughter in the emergency department. She came back in person to thank everyone for the care that was given to her mother and father.

## Studies and evidence about family presence

If the idea of FP is a totally new concept to a health care provider, it might be natural for some first thoughts to be about the potential emotional trauma and stress on family members during the event. This is a somewhat common belief until further investigation and review of the research literature about FP. There are at least three different types of research studies in the literature, and the sophisticated reader is encouraged to consider this schema in reviewing individual articles: (1) articles and surveys focused on provider fears, as expressed in individual beliefs and concerns about the notion of FP; (2) articles and surveys centered on provider what-ifs (eg, what if we tried this?); and (3) facts and evidence drawn from actual studies of the FP event and how various participants fared.

## Research about family members' experiences with family presence

A growing number of research studies demonstrate how the FP event affects family members and what they believe their roles to be. Numerous polls have been used to survey public opinions, including polls conducted by "NBC Dateline" [49] and *USA Today* [50], which showed a strong, majority (approximately 70%) sentiment in favor of staying with a loved one. A surprising number of studies have found that most family members want the option to be present during resuscitation and invasive procedures. Studies have described clearly the unique benefits of the experience to families, including (1) sustained patient-family connectedness and bonding [2,24], (2) sense of closure on a life shared together [2,8], (3) facilitation of the grief process [8,17, 20,23,25,27,28,51], (4) a spiritual experience [2], (5) removal of doubt about what is happening to the patient and knowledge that everything possible is being done [2,8,20,23,24,27,51], (6) reduced anxiety and fear [29,32,33,51], and (7) feeling of being supportive and helpful to the patient [2,8,24,26,27,29, 32,33]. Based on the findings from FP research, Doran [52] advocates that family members be offered a choice of being present in the ICU during brain stem death testing to facilitate acceptance of their loved one's death and promote the grieving process.

Health care providers opposed to FP often cite concerns about how families might interact during the resuscitation [9,53]. Researchers have found no disruptions in care provided by health care providers during FP events [2,8,17,23,25,27,30]. Robinson et al [51] stopped their randomized control trial of FP early because the staff said they were convinced of the benefits to families.

A qualitative study of the interactions among patients, families, and nurses in the trauma room also addressed the emotional responses of family members [54]. Morse and Pooler [54] recorded 193 scenarios with a video camera mounted to the wall in three Level I trauma centers in North American emergency departments. Family members were brought into the trauma room in 88 of the 193 cases. The length of time that families were at a patient's bedside varied from 20 seconds to 5 hours, with a mean time of 46 minutes. Families tended to enter the room after the most critical care and stabilization had been completed. By reviewing videotapes of the interactions, the researchers were able to describe common themes. Some family members manifested stoic behaviors, such as being silent or speaking only in short sentences. They tended to remain physically distant from the patient. Other family members displayed more emotional behaviors, including speaking consoling words to the patient or crying. These family members often were physically close to the patient or touched the patient in a caring manner. Most family members and patients displayed opposing reactions that countered each other. For example, when the patient became emotional, the family member became stoic. No family member lost control or interfered with medical care.

## Research about patients' experiences with family presence

Reports of patient attitudes regarding FP during resuscitation remain limited primarily because most do not survive the event. Robinson et al [51] reported on three patients who survived resuscitation who felt supported by their family's presence, and they did not feel that their privacy or dignity had been compromised. In the study by Eichhorn et al [55], 17 of 19 patients with attempted resuscitations died. This qualitative study reported on 9 patients who had families present during invasive procedures (8 in the emergency department) or CPR (1 in the ICU). Phone interviews were conducted 2 months after the emergency event to determine a patient's perceptions of FP. The interviews were done using a semi-structured questionnaire (the Family Presence Patient Interview Guide, developed by the researchers) and lasted an average of 45 minutes. Analysis revealed themes of patients receiving comfort from family members, family members acting as advocates, family members reminding the medical staff that the patient was a real person, increased connectedness to their family, and perception of FP as a right. These patients also acknowledged that FP was potentially stressful for their family members and that occasional limitations of the health care environment—such as space or family dynamics—could prevent FP from occurring. Overall, patients recognized that FP could be stressful for their families but believed that the benefits outweighed the risks.

Poor outcomes from resuscitation make the patient experience during FP difficult to study. Benjamin et al [56] administered a short survey about preferences should one ever need resuscitation to a convenience sample of patients and family members who were in an emergency department waiting room. Research assistants read a graphic resuscitation scenario to them (eg, "The patients are often naked," "Some bodily fluids, such as blood, urine, stool, may be present," and "cuts with a knife to put in chest tubes") and then asked questions. Of the 200 respondents, 72% responded favorably to having family members present during resuscitation; however, 56% of the positive responders wanted only certain family members to be present (54% wanted a spouse; 22% wanted siblings; 43% wanted parents; 31% wanted children; 22% wanted another person). Many subjects expressed a desire to have more than one family member present. Interviewees with negative responses to FP mentioned feelings of embarrassment that would possibly create painful lasting memories and fear of family getting in the way. The authors raised an interesting ethical question as to which is more important: the prestated wishes of patients, which may have occurred at a time when their own resuscitation seemed unlikely and were abstract ideaa, or the more beneficial and potentially long-lasting positive effects for the family members.

## Research about health care providers' experiences with family presence

Trends about health care providers that can be described after a decade of research include the premises that participating in FP alters one's perception of it after experiencing its feasibility and witnessing the benefits to families [10,11,20,25], nurses are more supportive of FP than physicians [2,9], and experienced physicians favor FP more than physicians in training [2,57]. Health care providers with actual experience with FP have supplied the most significant predictors of a supportive attitude [2,31].

Providing the option of FP should be delineated through written policies. These policies act as both a process description and a statement of the philosophy of the unit or hospital. Recently, MacLean et al [58] sent an anonymous survey to a random sample of 1500 nurses who were members of the American Association of Critical Care Nurses and 1500 members of the ENA. The purpose of the survey was to determine the preferences of critical care and emergency nurses and policies in reference to FP. Analysis of the 984 surveys returned revealed that only 5% of respondents worked on units that had formal written policies that allowed FP, but nearly half reported that their units allowed FP without a written policy. Thirty-six percent of these nurses had taken family members to the bedside during resuscitations, and 41% had allowed family members to be present during invasive procedures. In addition, 31% of respondents indicated that at least three families had approached them within the last year requesting to be present during CPR. Although most critical care and emergency nurses in this survey supported FP, approximately one third of the respondents indicated that they desired written policies allowing the option of FP. Because only 5% of the respondents worked on units with written policies, clearly there is a gap in relation to formalizing the process on paper.

Among nurses, educational levels and certification affect attitudes about FP. Ellison [59] compared the attitudes of 208 nurses who were either emergency department nurses or hospital nurses using the family presence support staff assessment survey. Researchers found that respondents who held certification as emergency nurses or had a Bachelor's or Master's degree had more positive attitudes about FP. Only 4% of nurses surveyed had ever attended an educational offering about FP. Overall, nurses who worked in the emergency department supported FP more than hospital nurses.

Generally, nurses and attending physicians in the emergency department were more supportive of FP than residents. Fein et al [57] surveyed 104 attending physicians, nurses, and pediatric medical residents working in a pediatric emergency department. Support for FP during medical and trauma resuscitation was similar among attending physicians and nurses (ranging from 62%–66%). Only 4% of pediatric medical residents supported FP during resuscitations. These trends were similar to results described in previous studies.

Two studies have described physician attitudes that contrast with others' findings about nurses. McClenathan et al [53] surveyed 592 attendees at the International Meeting of the American College of Chest Physicians in the year 2000, primarily adult critical care physicians, who did not reveal the same level of support in the ICU environment. Only 20% of physicians supported FP during adult resuscitations, and only 14% supported FP during pediatric resuscitations. The most common reasons cited for not supporting FP included psychological trauma to the family, increased anxiety and a fear of distraction among the CPR team, and medicolegal concerns. Helmer et al [9] reported a survey of 368 trauma surgeons and 1261 ENA members and found striking differences between the two groups. Nurses believed that FP was a patient and family right, and 64% reported positive feelings about it. Only 18% of physicians reported positive feelings, and many expressed concerns that it would interfere with CPR and increase litigation (rated 3.5/5, with 5 being "strongly agree").

## Finding family facilitators

Family members need to have a support person—or family facilitator—with them to prepare them for the experience, facilitate their placement in the room, tend to their needs, and help them deal with the likely outcome of resuscitation. The original Parkland Study was strengthened by use of a clinical nurse specialist with experience in trauma and psychosocial interventions [2]. Other possible sources of support for this role could come from various staff and volunteers, including social workers, chaplains, child life specialists, family therapists, nursing students, pharmacy students, and nurses who are interested in improving family-centered care [60]. An innovative role that is ideal for FP, called "clinical liaison nurse," is described in case study #3. Trained lay volunteers have been used successfully in many crisis situations, but reports of their use in FP have not been published [60].

The following narrative was written by a hospital chaplain who is currently part of an ongoing FP team. Two years before he became involved in FP, he started CPR on his father-in-law at home when he suffered a cardiac arrest, accompanied him with emergency medical services, and watched the resuscitation. He was the one who went to the emergency department waiting room and broke the news of the death to his wife and mother-in-law. He reported that from that moment, he was "haunted by the fact that I was there but my wife and her mother had to wait in another room. It never occurred to me to just go get them and bring them in" (Rev. Mike Norris, personal communication, 2004).

**Case #2: the Father Mulcahey effect**

The other night I was watching the old television sitcom series, "M*A*S*H," a show about an Army hospital in wartime Korea. In the episode, Father Francis Mulcahey, the unit chaplain, was writing a letter to his sister lamenting that he felt he was underused as a minister and chaplain among medical professionals. He had begun to notice that when intensive medical procedures were taking place, either in the operating room or the postsurgical ward, he felt he was an outsider—ministering on the periphery. He realized that all of the doctors, nurses, and medics were involved in saving the patient's life. He wrote in his letter that he had observed that during many of the lifesaving situations that happened at the M*A*S*H unit, he was just an observer.

Most of us who serve as hospital chaplains can relate to Father Mulcahey's lament, although it took place in a fictitious setting on a television show. Sometimes during code-blue and trauma situations it is difficult for spiritual caregivers to know their role. That was true for me, but I know when my thinking changed. It was when we began to do FP during CPR, traumas, and invasive procedures at our hospital. I am one of four staff chaplains who serve at our hospital, a 427-bed, level II trauma facility. When we decided to start FP, we made the decision to let families into CPR situations in the emergency department first before we implemented it as a hospital-wide policy. The idea was met with considerable resistance initially, especially from physicians concerned about litigation.

We did not realize in the beginning, however, how FP would change the way that spiritual care is done at our hospital and how we are viewed as spiritual caregivers. When a code blue is called in the emergency department—or on virtually all patient units (including all critical care units)—a chaplain responds with the code-blue team. The chaplain's job is to seek out the family members and explain what is happening in the room. We tell the family about the patient's situation, if we know it. In other words, we say, "Your husband has experienced a cardiac arrest." We make an assessment about how they can handle what they are going to see and offer them the chance to be present with their family member if they want to. We determine how much information the family members need before they go in. Above all, we make sure that they completely understand what is happening, which sometimes means telling them that they are going in to say goodbye.

FP has changed the way the staff sees the chaplain. Much of our work as chaplains is quiet and behind the scenes. We are called to anoint the sick, pray for people, and minister to families who are experiencing death and loss. Usually in these situations, nurses and physicians are busy with their own work and do not see what we do. Seeing us with the critical care team, helping the families, and being present at the critical moment has changed our relationships with the medical staff in positive ways that we did not expect. More importantly, this paradigm shift has caused us to see ourselves in a more positive light. We are part of the team that seeks to treat the whole family, and we are aware that our sacred duty is to be present. For the spiritual caregiver, the death of a patient is a critical, and yet sacred, moment.

**Recommendations for implementing a new family presence program**

Published confirmation of the value for FP is widely available in the literature and can lend support for health care providers who want to evaluate implementation. The ENA guidelines [44], "Presenting the Option for Family Presence," offer an excellent resource, including an extensive literature review, bibliography, slides, assessment instruments to evaluate the organization and staff readiness, liability issues, sample policy guidelines, and blueprints for implementation. Eichhorn et al [61] described the process of implementing FP in detail, including lessons learned and the importance of having a champion. This visionary leader can articulate the goal of FP to other leaders and health care providers and then move to institutionalize the vision [60,62]. The article by Meyers et al [2] contains the "Parkland Health and Hospital System: Protocol on Family Presence during Invasive Procedure and Resuscitation." McGahey [63] described FP pediatric issues, and a recent article by York [22] outlined useful steps to consider in planning. The article by Mangurten et al [45] detailed information about the processes to set up FP programs.

Several national authorities recommend FP and can shore up arguments to support FP initiatives in new settings. The recent "Guidelines 2000 for Cardiopulmonary Resuscitation and Emergency Cardiovascular Care" from the American Heart Association recommend that whenever possible, health care providers should offer family members the option to remain with their loved ones during resuscitation efforts [64]. This remarkable move was the first time that the American Heart Association included FP as a recommendation, and it has been a catalyst for many hospitals to evaluate its potential use [60]. The American Association of Critical Care Nurses identified FP as a priority for the organization and stated that all critical care units should have a written policy that allows the option of FP during invasive procedures and CPR [65]. FP is also recommended in the "Emergency Nursing Pediatric Course" [66] and the "Trauma Nurse Core Course" [67].

## Case #3: marketing family-centered care at your facility

The third case study of FP experience was written by a clinical liaison nurse, a unique emergency department staff nurse role developed to assist in all death-related circumstances, including miscarriages. Liaison nurses work closely with nurse colleagues. They carry the same certifications as other emergency department staff, are donor-requester qualified, and have attended bereavement classes. They report 10 AM to 10 PM as the most ideal hours, allowing for calls to physician offices when they are open and coverage into the busier evening hours. The follow-

ing case study was written by one of these nurses to describe her experience with FP.

I am present during many FP situations. One particular situation was moving and solidified my support and belief in FP. One afternoon, we received an ambulance patch on a patient who had collapsed from a cardiac arrest in her primary care physician's office less than a mile away from the hospital. When the patient arrived at our emergency department, CPR was in progress. The patient's husband followed, carrying his wife's purse. The look on his face was one of despair and fear.

As nurse liaison, I intercepted the husband and escorted him to the chest pain center to be at his wife's bedside. The patient had recently suffered a stroke, and her health had been deteriorating over the past month. Her sudden collapse in the doctor's office was a shock to everyone, however. When we entered the resuscitation room, the husband was given the option to stay. He chose to stay, and I explained what was happening during the attempted resuscitation. One of the patient's daughters soon arrived and was permitted into the room with the patient.

Resuscitation efforts continued, and the patient regained a pulse with a weak blood pressure. More family arrived, and the patient's daughters were all permitted to be at the bedside. The family was able to support each other and rotate in and out of the room as needed. The patient was transferred to the ICU but died shortly thereafter with her family at her side.

A month or so later, I received a beautiful thank you note from the patient's husband. In the midst of his grief, he was motivated to thank all who helped care for his wife during her last moments. He was deeply touched by the experience and felt that his wife received the best care possible. He saw everything that was done to save her life and felt that she was cared for with the utmost professionalism and compassion. He felt that this was by far the most supportive hospital experience that he had ever had.

I kept a copy of the letter and forwarded it to management. Months later, I was contacted by our director and asked if I would call the patient's husband to see if he would agree to be interviewed about his experience in FP. When I spoke to him, he was happy to be interviewed about a family member's perspective regarding FP. The husband again expressed his gratitude regarding his wife's entire resuscitation experience.

Soon afterward, he wrote this thank you letter to the staff:

> Please extend our thanks and appreciation for the kindness and efforts that were made to save my wife

and our mother. We wish we could thank everybody individually but our memories did not allow us to remember names of all those who gave the extra effort to save her. A special thank you to the doctors and nurses in the emergency and ICU, and the chaplain. The courtesies extended to myself, daughters, son-in-law, grandchildren are unequaled. The warmth and kindness we received during our time of grief and loss was unequalled by any other hospital experience. You are all to be commended for that extra effort that was felt by all of us. Thank you, and may God bless you all.

## Summary

Caring for families in crisis remains a challenge for health care providers. Allowing family members to remain with their loved one during resuscitation events, if they desire, offers them potential benefits in supporting the grief process and facilitating coping and understanding what was done to treat the patient. Despite predictions by some, FP has shown to be well tolerated by family members who feel an emotional connection with their loved one that continues until death. Family members always should be accompanied by someone who focuses on their needs and allows persons involved in the resuscitation event itself to direct their undivided attention to the task at hand. When available, chaplains (including students and community minister volunteers) who are skilled in counseling and support should join FP teams. Multiple resources are available to leaders who are considering FP programs as a part of improving family-centered care.

Berwick and Kotagal [68] recently wrote in the *Journal of the American Medical Association* that available evidence shows that hazards and problems with open visitation in the ICU are generally overstated and manageable. They suggest testing an unrestricted visiting hour policy for a few months and then reflecting on the successes and obstacles actually experienced. The result will be "better patient- and family-centered care for those patients who are most in need." We believe that FP is a logical extension of this family-centered culture and deserves our consideration.

## References

[1] Henneman EA, Cardin S. Family-centered critical care: a practical approach to making it happen. Crit Care Nurse 2002;22(6):12–9.

[2] Meyers TA, Eichhorn DJ, Guzzetta CE, et al. Family presence during invasive procedures and resuscitation. Am J Nurs 2000;100(2):32–42.

[3] Bauchner H, Vinci R, Waring C. Pediatric procedures: do parents want to watch? Pediatrics 1989;84: 907–9.

[4] Boudreaux ED, Francis JL, Loyacano T. Family presence during invasive procedures and resuscitations in the emergency department: a critical review and suggestions for future research. Ann Emerg Med 2002; 40(2):193–205.

[5] Boyd R, White S. Does witnessed cardiopulmonary resuscitation alter perceived stress in accident and emergency staff? Eur J Emerg Med 1998;7(1):51–3.

[6] Chalk A. Should relatives be present in the resuscitation room? Accid Emerg Nurs 1995;3(2):58–61.

[7] Fiorentini SE. Evaluation of a new program: pediatric parental visitation in the postanesthesia care unit. J Post Anesth Nurs 1993;8:249–56.

[8] Hanson C, Strawser D. Family presence during cardiopulmonary resuscitation: Foote Hospital emergency department's nine-year perspective. J Emerg Nurs 1992;18:104–6.

[9] Helmer SD, Smith RS, Dort JM, et al. Family presence during trauma resuscitation: a survey of AAST and ENA members. J Trauma 2000;48(6):1015–20.

[10] Jarvis AS. Parental presence during resuscitation: attitudes of staff on a paediatric intensive care unit. Intensive Crit Care Nurs 1998;4(1):3–7.

[11] Mitchell MH, Lynch MB. Should relatives be allowed in the resuscitation room? J Accid Emerg Med 1997; 14(6):366–9.

[12] Post H. Letting the family in during a code. Nursing 1989;89:43–6.

[13] Proehl JA, Smith SS. Point/counterpoint: should family members be present during codes? Phys Weekly 2000;17(18):1.

[14] Redheffer GM. A trauma nurse's opinion [commentary]. Nursing 1989;89:45.

[15] Redley B, Hood K. Staff attitudes towards family presence during resuscitation. Accid Emerg Nurs 1996; 4(3):145–51.

[16] Reynolds D. Death as a shared experience. ED Management 1992;14(2):177–81.

[17] Sacchetti A, Lichenstein R, Carraccio CA, et al. Family member presence during pediatric emergency department procedures. Pediatr Emerg Care 1996; 12(4):268–71.

[18] Sanford M, Pugh D, Warren NA. Family presence during CPR: new decisions in the twenty-first century. Crit Care Nurs Q 2002;25(2):61–6.

[19] Taylor N, Bonilla L, Silver P, et al. Pediatric procedures: do parents want to be present? Crit Care Med 1996;24(Suppl):131.

[20] Timmermans S. High touch in high tech: the presence of relatives and friends during resuscitation efforts. Sch Inq Nurs Pract 1997;11:153–68.

[21] Tucker TL. Family presence during resuscitation. Crit Care Nurs Clin North Am 2002;14:177–85.

[22] York NL. Implementing a family presence protocol option. Dimens Crit Care Nurs 2004;23(2):84–8.

[23] Anderson B, McCall E, Leversha A, et al. A review of children's dying in a paediatric intensive care unit. N Z Med J 1985;107:345–7.

[24] Bauchner H, Waring C, Vinci R. Parental presence during procedures in an emergency room: results from 50 observations. Pediatrics 1991;87:544–8.

[25] Belanger MA, Reed S. A rural community hospital's experience with family-witnessed resuscitation. J Emerg Nurs 1997;23(3):238–9.

[26] Berns R, Colvin ER. The final story: events at the bedside of dying patients as told by survivors. ANNA J 1998;25:583–7.

[27] Doyle CJ, Post H, Burney RE, et al. Family participation during resuscitation: an option. Ann Emerg Med 1987;16:673–5.

[28] Meyers TA, Eichhorn DJ, Guzzetta CE. Do families want to be present during CPR? A retrospective survey. J Emerg Nurs 1998;24:400–5.

[29] Powers KS, Rubenstein JS. Family presence during invasive procedures in the pediatric intensive care unit. Arch Pediatr Adolesc Med 1999;153:955–8.

[30] Robinson CA. Beyond dichotomies in the nursing of persons and families. Image (IN) 1995;27(2):116–9.

[31] Sacchetti A, Carraccio C, Leva E, et al. Acceptance of family member presence during pediatric resuscitation in the emergency department: effects of personal experience. Pediatr Emerg Care 2000;16(2):85–7.

[32] Shapira M, Tamir A. Presence of family member during upper endoscopy. J Clin Gastroenterol 1996;22: 272–4.

[33] Turner P. Establishing a protocol for parental presence in recovery. Br J Nurs 1997;6(14):794, 796–9.

[34] Peberdy MA, Kaye W, Ornato JP, et al, for the NRCPR Investigators. Cardiopulmonary resuscitation of adults in the hospital: a report of 14,720 cardiac arrests from the National Registry of Cardiopulmonary Resuscitation. Resuscitation 2003;58:297–308.

[35] Stiell IG, Wells GA, Field BJ, et al. Improved out-of-hospital cardiac arrest survival through the inexpensive optimization of an existing defibrillation program: OPALS study phase II. JAMA 1999;281(13):1175–81.

[36] Van Walraven C, Forster AJ, Stiell IG. Derivation of a clinical decision rule for the discontinuation of in-hospital cardiac arrest resuscitations. Arch Intern Med 1999;159:129–34.

[37] Auble TE, Menegazzi JJ, Paris PM. Effect of out-of-hospital defibrillation by basic life support providers on cardiac arrest mortality: a metaanalysis. Ann Emerg Med 1995;25:642–8.

[38] Timmermans S. Sudden death and the myth of CPR. Philadelphia: Temple University Press; 1999. p. 31–89.

[39] Kouwenhoven WB, Jude JR, Knickerbocker GG. Closed chest cardiac massage. JAMA 1960;173: 1064–7.

[40] Public Access Defibrillation Trial Investigators. Public-access defibrillation and survival after out-of-hospital cardiac arrest. N Engl J Med 2004;351:637–46.

[41] Stiell IG, Wells GA, Field B, et al. Advanced cardiac life support in out-of-hospital cardiac arrest. N Engl J Med 2004;351:647–56.

[42] Joglar JA, Page RL. Cardiopulmonary resuscitation: modern improvements on basic life support. In: Crawford MH, DiMarco JP, Paulus WJ, editors. Cardiology. 2nd edition. Edinburgh: Mosby; 2004. p. 787–95.

[43] Emergency Nurses Association. Presenting the option for family presence [program educational booklet]. Park Ridge (IL): The Association; 1995. p. 1–84.

[44] Emergency Nurses Association. Presenting the option for family presence [program educational booklet]. Des Plaines (IL): The Association; 2001. p. 1–87.

[45] Mangurten J, Scott S, Guzzetta C, et al. Changing conventional practice: implementing family presence during resuscitation interventions and invasive procedure. Am J Nurs, in press.

[46] Van Horn E, Fleury J, Moore S. Family interventions during the trajectory of recovery from cardiac event: an integrative literature review. Heart Lung 2002;31(3): 186–98.

[47] Kirchhoff K, Walker L, Hutton A, et al. The vortex: families' experience with death in the intensive care unit. Am J Crit Care 2002;11(3):200–9.

[48] Merlevede E, Spooren D, Henderick H, et al. Perceptions, needs and mourning reactions of bereaved relatives confronted with a sudden unexpected death. Resuscitation 2004;61:341–8.

[49] Should family members of patients be allowed in the ED during emergency procedures? [poll]. Available at: http://www.dateline.msnbc.com. Accessed August 6, 1999.

[50] Would you want to be in the ED while doctors worked on a family member? [poll]. Available at: http://www.USATODAY.com Accessed March 7, 2000.

[51] Robinson SM, Mackenzie-Ross S, Campbell-Hewson GL, et al. Psychological effect of witnessed resuscitation on bereaved relatives. Lancet 1998;352:614–7.

[52] Doran M. The presence of family during brain stem death testing. Intensive Crit Care Nurs 2004; 20(1):32–7.

[53] McClenathan BM, Torrington KG, Uyehara CFT. Family member presence during cardiopulmonary resuscitation: a survey of US and international critical care professionals. Chest 2002;122:2204–11.

[54] Morse JM, Pooler C. Patient-family-nurse interactions in the trauma-resuscitation room. Am J Crit Care 2002; 11:240–9.

[55] Eichhorn DJ, Meyers TA, Guzzetta CE, et al. Family presence during invasive procedures and resuscitation: hearing the voice of the patient. Am J Nurs 2001; 101(5):26–33.

[56] Benjamin M, Holder J, Carr M. Personal preferences regarding family member presence during resuscitation. Acad Emerg Med 2004;11:750–3.

[57] Fein JA, Ganesh J, Alpern ER. Medical staff attitudes toward family presence during pediatric procedures. Pediatr Emerg Care 2004;20:224–7.

[58] MacLean SL, Guzzetta CE, White C, et al. Family presence during cardiopulmonary resuscitation and invasive procedures: practices of critical care and emergency nurses. Am J Crit Care 2003;12:246–57.

[59] Ellison S. Nurses' attitudes toward family presence during resuscitative efforts and invasive procedures. J Emerg Nurs 2003;29:515–21.

[60] Clark AP, Calvin AO, Meyers TA, et al. Family presence during cardiopulmonary resuscitation and invasive procedures: a research-based intervention. Crit Care Nurs Clin North Am 2001;13:569–75.

[61] Eichhorn DJ, Meyers TA, Guzzetta CE, et al. Family presence at the bedside during invasive procedures and CPR: when pigs fly. In: Mason DJ, Leavitt JK, editors. Policy and politics in nursing and health care. 4th edition. Philadelphia: WB Saunders; 2002.

[62] Ulschak FL, Snow Antle SM. Team architecture: the manager's guide to designing effective work teams. Ann Arbor: Health Administration Press; 1997.

[63] McGahey PR. Family presence during pediatric resuscitation: a focus on staff. Crit Care Nurs 2002; 22(6):29–34.

[64] American Heart Association, in Collaboration with the International Liaison Committee on Resuscitation. Guidelines 2000 for cardiopulmonary resuscitation and emergency cardiovascular care. Circulation 2000; 102(8 Suppl):I-374.

[65] Knight KA. Intensive caring: 24/7 access in the ICU. Available at: http://community.nursingspectrum.com/ MagazineArticles/article.cfm?AID=11204. Accessed March 22, 2004.

[66] Eckle N, Haley K, Baker P, editors. Emergency nursing pediatric course: provider manual. 2nd edition. Park Ridge (IL): The Emergency Nurses Association; 1998. p. 70, 141.

[67] Jacobs BB, Hoyt KS, editors. Trauma nursing core course: provider manual. 5th edition. Park Ridge (IL): The Emergency Nurses Association; 2000. p. 47, 290–1.

[68] Berwick DM, Kotagal M. Restricted visiting hours in ICUs: time to change. JAMA 2004;292(6): 736–7.

ELSEVIER
SAUNDERS

Crit Care Nurs Clin N Am 17 (2005) 33–38

CRITICAL CARE
NURSING CLINICS
OF NORTH AMERICA

# Clinical Trials Update: Sudden Cardiac Death Prevention by Implantable Device Therapy

## Nancy J. Finch, RN, PhD[a],*, Robert B. Leman, MD[b]

[a]*College of Nursing, Medical University of South Carolina, 99 Jonathan Lucas Street, PO Box 250160,
Charleston, SC 29425, USA*
[b]*Department of Medicine, Medical University of South Carolina, 135 Rutledge Avenue, Suite 1201, Charleston, SC 29425, USA*

Sudden cardiac death represents an enormous public health problem in all developed countries of the world. In the United States, sudden cardiac death occurs in more than 400,000 people each year and is the leading cause of death. In sudden cardiac death, the heart abruptly and unexpectedly ceases to function (cardiac arrest), presumably because of an electrical disturbance. Individuals deemed high risk for sudden cardiac death may be treated with implantable defibrillators. This article highlights evidence from randomized, controlled trials of implantable device therapy used in prevention of sudden cardiac death.

## Sudden cardiac death

Sudden cardiac death (SCD) is the abrupt natural death that is unexpected and occurs within a brief time period (less than 1–12 hours) depending on the study used to define it. SCD, a major health problem throughout the world, is seen in the United States in approximately 400,000 to 450,000 people each year and around the world in approximately 3 million people [1,2]. SCD gets little notoriety, perhaps because it is short lived, although it affects more lives than a multiple of other diseases. SCD claims more lives than a combination of throat, lung, or breast cancer and AIDS [1,3]. In 1999, only the total mortality from all cancers combined had a higher mor-

tality in the general population than SCD [2,4]. The cause of SCD has been linked clearly to coronary disease, which is present in approximately 80% of victims. The second most common cause is cardiomyopathy, which occurs in 10% to 15%. The incidence of sudden death could be decreased by eliminating coronary disease entirely. Although great strides have been made in improving the incidence of coronary artery disease (CAD) in social and medical therapies, the incidence still continues to be a problem. Primary and secondary prevention of SCD, the focus of this article, becomes increasingly important.

## Primary and secondary prevention

Therapeutic strategies for the prevention of SCD are divided into two general categories: primary and secondary prevention. The term "primary" as it relates to the prevention of SCD is at variance with the conventional definition of primary prevention, which refers to prevention of the underlying disease. By definition and usage in the arrhythmia field, "primary" has come to mean prevention of the first potentially fatal arrhythmic event [5].

Secondary prevention in this field is used to describe prevention of a recurrence of a potentially fatal arrhythmia or cardiac arrest among patients who have had a prior event. Within each category, the most common anti-arrhythmic strategies have been pharmacologic and implantable cardioverter defibrillators (ICDs) [5].

---

\* Corresponding author.
*E-mail address:* finchn@musc.edu (N.J. Finch).

## Populations at risk for sudden cardiac death

The definition of SCD as being a natural event is probably the result of the asymptomatic status of people with underlying disease processes and the fact that the frequency is uncommon in the general population—approximately 0.1% and 0.2% [6]. Whereas the incidence is low, the total number of people affected is large because it includes the whole population. If other morbidity factors are included, such as low ejection fraction (EF), cardiac arrest survival, myocardial infarction, and high-risk myocardial infarction patients, the incidence of SCD rises dramatically to 20% to 30%. Whereas the incidence is higher, the total number of patients affected is smaller because of the group size. We must target patients with CAD as a primary entity to help decrease the incidence of sudden death. Heart failure (HF) also has a major effect on the incidence of sudden death, which has been shown to increase from 1.4% in persons with a more than 50% EF to 7.5% in persons with a less than 30% EF [7]. Several interventions have improved the sensitivity and specificity by adding various comorbidities.

Because the primary cause of sudden death is CAD, patients with this disease must be evaluated more closely. It is known that approximately 1.1 million heart attacks occur annually, which accounts for a total population in the United States of 12 million people who have CAD [8]. If one considers

persons with CAD and an EF of 30%, there would be approximately 405,000 patients a year who would qualify to be in this high-risk group [9]. SCD has not only a high mortality problem but also a low survival rate, even if found early. Unfortunately, the overall survival rate of patients with SCD is dismal—only 5% in the United States and 1% in the rest of the world [10]. The benefit of treatment is greater in primary prevention than secondary.

The problem with the primary prevention of sudden death is the difficulty in determining individuals at risk, other than the population of patients with coronary disease and HF. Unfortunately in the general population, coronary disease and cardiac dysfunction are often subclinical or unknown. The initial studies that focused on prevention of sudden death were actually the secondary prevention trials.

## Secondary prevention trials with sudden cardiac death

Table 1 displays three treatment trials that examined secondary prevention of aborted SCD or syncope believed to be secondary to ventricular arrhythmias. These trials were conducted at a time when anti-arrhythmic therapy was believed to be adequate treatment and compared that treatment with the newer ICDs. The three trials, the AVID (Anti-arrhythmic vs Implantable Defibrillator Trial), the

Table 1
Secondary prevention trial for patients with aborted sudden cardiac death or syncope (implantable cardioverter defibrillators) compared to antiarrhythmic drugs

|  | Study | | |
|  | AVID | CASH | CIDS |
| --- | --- | --- | --- |
| Year | 2002 | 2004 | 2004 |
| No. of patients | 1016 | 288 | 659 |
| % CAD | 81% | 77% | 83% |
| CHF Class I | 40%–45% | 23%–32% | 49%–51% |
| II | 48% | 55%–59% | 37%–40% |
| III | 7%–12% | 13%–18% | 10%–11% |
| IV |  | 0 |  |
| Inclusion EF | <40% | Not applicable | ≤35% |
| Mean EF | 32% | 46% | 34% |
| Medications | Amiodarone | Amiodarone | Amiodarone |
|  | Sotalol | Propafenone, metoprolol | Amiodarone |
| Follow-up | 1.5 y | 4.75 y | 3 y |
| Relative risk reduction | 31% | 23% | 20% |
|  | $P < 0.02$ | $P = 0.081$ | $P = 0.142$ |
|  | If EF >34% |  |  |
|  | $P$ not significant |  |  |

*Abbreviations*: AVID, anti-arrhythmic versus implantable defibrillator; CAD, coronary artery disease; CASH, cardiac arrest study Hamburg; CHF, congestive heart failure; CIDS, Canadian implant defibrillator study; EF, ejection fraction.

CASH (Cardiac Arrest Study Hamburg Trial), and the CIDS (Canadian Implant Defibrillator Trial), compared ICD treatment with various medications. The primary medication in all of these trials was amiodarone. These trials reported an incidence of coronary disease of approximately 80%. Cardiac function was abnormal, although in the CASH trial it was not as low as currently believed to be necessary.

In the comparative trials, CASH had three drug therapies; one drug was stopped early (Propafenone) secondary to adverse events. Each of these trials showed that the reduction of sudden death was improved by ICD implantation over drug therapy. The relative risk reduction, although in favor of the ICD, was not statistically different in the CASH trial or the CIDS trial, however. The reduction of sudden death was not significant for the AVID trial for patients with an EF of more than 34%. Initially the AVID trial, which was the largest, showed the significance of ICD therapy in the overall trial, and in patients with an EF of less than 34% it showed a benefit. Further trials were initiated to look for primary prevention of sudden death by ICD therapy.

## Primary prevention trials with coronary artery disease

Table 2 examines three primary prevention trials in patients with CAD. These three trials included patients with known CAD. The MADIT I (Multicenter Automatic Defibrillator Implantation Trial) and the MUSTT (Multicenter Unsustained Tachycar-

dia Trial) had inclusion criteria of a nonsustained ventricular tachycardia and an EF of less than 35% or 40%, depending on the trial. Patients had to be inducible into a ventricular arrhythmia by electrophysiologic study. The CABG PATCH trial examined patients who underwent coronary artery bypass surgery for ischemic heart disease and had an inclusion criterion of a positive signal averaging electrocardiogram with an EF of less than 36%. The results of the MADIT I and MUSTT were impressive because of a significant reduction in the subset of patients who were believed to be at high risk. Their relative risk reduction ranged from 51% to 54% depending on the trial and was statistically significant to a $P$ value of 0.001 or 0.009. The CABG PATCH trial did not show a reduction of sudden death, however. The difference was that the CABG PATCH trial had no inclusion of ventricular arrhythmias or inducible arrhythmias in its group. It becomes clear by the MADIT I and MUSTT trials that a subset of patients with CAD, nonsustained ventricular tachycardia, and a positive Electrophysiologic study clearly benefit significantly and have a marked reduction of mortality with ICD implantation. Unfortunately, the group that qualifies for this is not large, and fewer inclusion criteria were used to improve or expand the number of patients protected by ICD therapy.

## Primary prevention trials with heart failure

The diagnosis of HF is another factor shown to affect survival in persons with and without CAD.

Table 2
Primary prevention trials with coronary artery disease

|  | Study | | |
|---|---|---|---|
|  | MADIT I | MUSTT | CABG Patch |
| Year | 1996 | 1999 | 1997 |
| No. of patients | 196 | 704 | 900 |
| % CAD | 100% | 100% | 100% |
| CHF Class I | 33%–37% | 36%–37% | ? |
| II | 63%–67% | 38%–39% | 71%–74% |
| III |  | 24%–25% |  |
| IV | 0 | 0 | ? |
| Inclusion | NSVT, EPS | NSVT, EPS | SAE |
| EF inclusion | ≤35% | ≥40% | <36% |
| Mean EF | ~26% | ~30% | ~27% |
| Follow-up | 2.25 y | 3.25 y | 2.66 y |
| Relative risk reduction | 54% | 51% | Nonsignificant |
|  | $P = 0.009$ | $P < 0.001$ |  |

*Abbreviations:* CABG Patch, coronary artery bypass graft patch trial; EPS, electrophysiologic study; MADIT I, multicenter automatic defibrillator implantation trial; MUSTT, multicenter unsustained tachycardia trial; NSVT, nonsustained ventricular tachycardia; SAE, signal averaging electrocardiogram.

Three trials have addressed the issue of HF as a main cause for risk stratification in treatment with ICD therapy: the MADIT II trial (Multicenter Automatic Defibrillator Implantation Trial II), the SCDHeFT trial (Sudden Cardiac Death and Heart Failure Trial), and the DEFINITE trial (Defibrillators in Nonischemic Cardiomyopathy Treatment Evaluation) as noted in Table 3. These trials were the first to include nonischemic cardiomyopathy. The MADIT II trial was a CAD trial, the SCDHeFT trial included 48% nonischemic cardiomyopathies, and the DEFINITE trial included only nonischemic cardiomyopathies. For all three trials, only patients with EFs less than 30% to 36% were included. They had no further inclusion for ventricular arrhythmias. Criteria included only HF and EF. Each of these trials was relatively large except for the DEFINITE trial. All of the trials showed a relative risk reduction from 23% to 35%.

The DEFINITE trial, which was a smaller trial, was not statistically significant for overall mortality. It was statistically significant for a reduction of sudden death, however. There was a decrease in the incidence from medical treatment of 6.1% to ICD treatment of 1.3%, with a $P$ value of 0.006. The other trials (MADIT II and SCDHeFT), however, did show a statistical reduction in SCD ICD implantation. A substudy of the MADIT II patients used width of the QRS as an additional selection filter. The analysis revealed that (1) patients with a QRS more than 120 msec were found to have a 63% relative reduction of mortality to a $P$ value of 0.004, (2) patients

with a QRS more than or equal to 120 msec were found to have a risk reduction of 49% with a $P$ value of 0.07, and (3) patients with a QRS of less than 120 msec and a risk reduction of approximately 25% were found to be similar to the overall results [11].

Just looking at the EF, the primary prevention trials again showed statistically improved survival with ICD therapy. Relative risk reduction is not as impressive as the trials (MADIT I and MUSTT) that were more restrictive and included nonsustained ventricular tachycardia and electrophysiologic study induction of ventricular arrhythmias. By using these trials, however, one can further improve or extend the survival benefit of ICD therapy to a greater population. The question then becomes whether there is a better way to subselect and target patients who truly need ICD therapy and eliminate some of the less effective implantations.

### Linking research to practice

Because of these findings, the American College of Cardiology, the American Heart Association, and the North American Society of Pacing and Electrophysiology have made several changes to the 2002 guidelines for implantation of cardiac pacemakers and ICDs.

The American College of Cardiology and American Heart Association classifications for I and II indications for ICD implantation are defined as follows:

Class I: Conditions for which there is evidence or general agreement that a given procedure or treatment is useful and effective.

Class II: Conditions for which there is conflicting evidence or a divergence of opinion about the usefulness or efficacy of a procedure or treatment.

Class IIa: Weight of evidence or opinion is in favor of usefulness and efficacy.

Class IIb: Usefulness and efficacy are less well established by evidence or opinion [12].

One of the specific recommendations comes from the MADIT II trial, which states that patients with left ventricular EFs of less than or equal to 30% at least 1 month after myocardial infarction and 3 months after coronary bypass surgery are designated as a Class IIa indication for ICD implantation. An additional ICD implant recommendation is seen in patients with syncope with advanced structural heart disease in whom a thorough investigation—invasive and non-

Table 3
Primary prevention trials with congestive heart failure

|  | Study | | |
|---|---|---|---|
|  | MADIT II | SCDHeFT | DEFINITE |
| Year | 2002 | 2004 | 2004 |
| No. of patients | 1232 | 2521 | 458 |
| % CAD | 100% | 52% | 0% |
| Class CHF inclusion | I–III | II–III | I–III |
| Class I | 35%–39% | O | 21.6% |
| II | 34%–35% | 70% | 57.4% |
| III | 23%–25% | 30% | 21% |
| IV | 4%–5% | 0 | 0 |
| EF inclusion | <30% | ≤35% | <36% |
| EF mean | 23% | 25% | 21% |
| Follow-up | 1.67 y | 2.5 y | 2.42 y |
| Relative risk reduction | 31% $P$ = 0.016 | 23% $P$ = 0.007 | 35% $P$ = 0.08 |

*Abbreviations*: DEFINITE, defibrillators in nonischemic cardiomyopathy treatment evaluation; MADIT II, multicenter automatic defibrillator implantation trial II; SCDHeFT, sudden cardiac death and heart failure trial.

invasive—failed to find a definitive cause. They are designated as a Class IIb. These two recommendations show that the primary prevention studies on HF had significant input in changing the indications for ICDs.

Unfortunately, Medicare reimbursement has not followed these guidelines and still allows coverage only for patients who meet the criteria of EF of less than 30%, CAD, and a wide QRS complex on electrocardiogram. Although we can conclude that EFs are probably the most important indicators for ICD implantation followed by the presence of CAD and wide QRSs, we should continue to search for other markers that can improve the effectiveness, sensitivity, and specificity of ICD implantation.

**Implications for clinical practice**

The challenges presented to health care practitioners are uniquely complex. How does one translate the results of randomized, controlled trials into daily clinical practice with individual patients? Existing evidence of ICD efficacy in specific subsets of patients for primary and secondary prevention of SCD has been discussed (Tables 1–3).

The MADIT I and MUSTT trials showed that the ICDs improved survival in high-risk patients with CAD when compared with conventional medical therapy. The MADIT II trial showed that prophylactic ICD therapy significantly improved survival in patients with ischemic cardiomyopathy, as defined by documented CAD and advanced left ventricular dysfunction, without screening for ventricular arrhythmias or inducibility by electrophysiologic study testing [13].

The most recent findings from the SCDHeFT trial showed a clinically and statistically significant benefit from ICDs implanted in patients with HF with a left ventricular EF of less than or equal to 35%. These data recently were presented at the American College of Cardiology by the primary investigators (March 8, 2004). Publication of the SCDHeFT data is expected by the end of the year. Clinical research has demonstrated that ICDs are safe and effective in primary and secondary prevention of SCD, and knowledge of the selection criteria used in clinical trials guides practitioners in the identification of patients who will receive the most benefit from ICD therapy.

**Implications for community practice**

The challenges presented to health care providers in community practice are equally important. Myerburg et al [14] reviewed the issue of the risk of SCD in population subgroups and their contribution to the overall burden of SCD. Asymptomatic individuals with multiple risk factors for coronary disease are at higher risk than the population at large, whereas individuals with known cardiac disease pathology are at even greater risk. Developing coronary risk factor screening tools that are reliable facilitates identification of individuals who are at the highest risk. Differentiating the categories (high-risk versus low-risk groups) determines the level of management. Consultation and referral to electrophysiology cardiologists for further evaluation and treatment are essential.

Perhaps the greatest challenge lies in identifying potential victims of SCD in the population of lower risk individuals. Even people who appear healthy and free of heart disease can experience arrhythmias. Because the underlying cause of an arrhythmia is not always clear, the best course of action is preventing and delaying their development. Arrhythmia prevention includes preventing heart disorders in general, including eliminating risk factors that may lead to cardiovascular disease or cardiac arrhythmias. Making healthy lifestyle choices is the best way to decrease the chances of developing heart disorders. Providing risk factor screening and education about prevention is the responsibility of all health care providers.

**Implications for primary and secondary prevention**

Primary prevention for ventricular fibrillation and SCD may include (1) adopting a "heart healthy" lifestyle that includes regular exercise and a low fat diet, maintaining ideal body weight, and stopping or avoiding smoking, (2) treating and monitoring underlying diseases, such as hypertension and diabetes, (3) diagnosing and correcting arrhythmias, and (4) instituting prophylactic treatment with ICD implantation in high-risk groups [15], such as persons who meet MADIT II and SCDHeFT eligibility criteria. Secondary preventions for ventricular fibrillation and SCD may include the implantation of an ICD with or without the addition of an anti-arrhythmic agent [15].

**Implications for research and policy**

Research dissemination to all health care providers and payers is critical to enhance their knowledge of the effectiveness of using implantable defibrillators for prevention of SCD. The Heart Rhythm Society (formally North American Society of Pacing and Electrophysiology) has submitted a statement to the Centers for Medicare and Medicaid Services that supports full coverage of the SCDHeFT patient population trial [16]. It is anticipated that the Centers for Medicare and Medicaid Services will publish a draft decision by September 30, 2004. A 30-day comment period will follow, and the earliest that a final decision is expected is December 30, 2004 (Amy Melnick, personal communication, 2004).

In February 2005, the Heart Rhythm Foundation will launch its first public and patient awareness campaign directed at persons at risk for SCD. The program initially will be piloted in Minnesota and will target individuals who have had a coronary event (eg, myocardial infarction, cardiac arrest, or HF). A screening will be offered that includes an echocardiogram to measure EF and an electrocardiogram. Educational awareness about SCD and its treatment will be provided to the community of health care providers. An evaluation of the campaign and an analysis of the outcomes data will be reported at the Heart Rhythm Foundation annual sessions in May 2005 (Lisa Olson, PhD, personal communication, 2004).

## Summary

SCD remains a major public health issue. Real progress in reducing its impact depends on identification of individuals at risk and reduction of those risk factors through education, screening, and treatment. The application of research findings from randomized clinical trials using ICDs for primary and secondary prevention of SCD has shown safety and efficacy. Selecting the most effective treatments based on clinical research leads to improved survival and a reduction in SCD mortality. Ongoing support of clinical trials research should continue to advance the knowledge and science of practice. Linking research findings to policymaking is essential to the development of public health policy. The greatest challenges will be in global prevention efforts that require the commitment of all medical and public health researchers and clinicians working together to improve methods to identify and treat persons at risk for SCD.

## Acknowledgments

The authors would like to extend a special thanks to Suzanne Gresle, MA, MS, and Jeanie Poore for their contributions in the preparation of this article.

## References

[1] Zheng ZJ, Croft JB, Giles WH, et al. Sudden cardiac death in the United States, 1989 to 1998. Circulation 2001;104(18):2158–63.

[2] Centers for Disease Control and Prevention. State-specific mortality from sudden cardiac death: United States, 1999. MMWR Morb Mortal Wkly Rep 2002; 51(6):123–6.

[3] Census Bureau. Statistical abstract of the United States, 2002. American Cancer Society surveillance research: Cancer facts and figures 2001.

[4] Anderson RN. Deaths: leading causes for 1999. National vital statistics reports. Hyattsville (MD): National Center for Health Statistics; 2001. p. 1–88.

[5] Myerburg RJ, Spooner PM. Opportunities for sudden death prevention: directions for new clinical and basic research. Cardiovasc Res 2001;50:177–85.

[6] Myerburg RJ. Sudden cardiac death: exploring the limits of our knowledge. J Cardiovasc Electrophysiol 2001;12:369–81.

[7] de-Vreede-Swagemakers JJ, Gorgels AP, Dubois-Arbouw WI, et al. Out-of-hospital cardiac arrest in the 1990s: a population-based study in the Maastricht area on incidence, characteristics and survival. J Am Coll Cardiol 1997;30(6):1500–5.

[8] American Heart Association. 2002 Heart and Stroke Statistical Update. Dallas (TX): American Heart Association; 2002.

[9] Bigger JT, Fleiss JL, Kleiger R, et al. The relationships among ventricular arrhythmias, left ventricular dysfunction and mortality in the two years after myocardial infarction. Circulation 1984;69:250–8.

[10] Myerburg RJ, Catellanos A. Cardiac arrest and sudden cardiac death. In: Braunwald E, editor. Heart disease: a textbook of cardiovascular medicine. 5th edition. Philadelphia: WB Saunders; 1997. p. 742–79.

[11] Zareba W. Late breaking clinical trials: noninvasive electrocardiology and outcome in MADIT II patients. Presented at NASPE Annual Sessions. May 11, 2002.

[12] American College of Cardiology/American Heart Association Task Force on Practice Guidelines. Practice guidelines update for implantation of cardiac pacemakers and antiarrhythmia devices. Circulation 2002;106:2145–61.

[13] Moss AJ. MADIT-I and MADIT-II review. J Cardiovasc Electrophysiol 2003;14(9 Suppl):S96–8.

[14] Myerburg RJ, Kessler KM, Castellanos A. Sudden cardiac death: structure, function, and time-dependence of risk. Circulation 1992;81(1 Suppl):I2–10.

[15] Heart Rhythm Society. Sudden cardiac death (cardiac arrest) prevention. Available at: http://www.hrspatients.org/patients/heart_disorders/cardiac_arrest/prevention.asp. Accessed July 23, 2004.

[16] NASPE, Heart Rhythm Society. Washington report: SCDHeFT. April 28, 2004. Available at: http://www.naspe@NASPE.org.

ELSEVIER
SAUNDERS

Crit Care Nurs Clin N Am 17 (2005) 39 – 43

CRITICAL CARE
NURSING CLINICS
OF NORTH AMERICA

# Documentation of Resuscitation Events

## Patricia Kunz Howard, PhD, RN, CEN[a,b,*]

[a]Cardiovascular Nursing, College of Nursing, University of Kentucky, Lexington, KY 40536-0232, USA
[b]Emergency Department, University of Kentucky Hospital, Lexington, KY, USA

Documentation is an integral aspect of nursing. The well-known phrase "if it wasn't documented, it never happened" aptly describes the importance of documentation. Resuscitation events are a potential documentation nightmare, with many events occurring nearly simultaneously and multiple personnel involved. Documentation of resuscitation events is essential to determining what care was actually provided during the event, critically evaluating how a patient responded to resuscitation interventions, ensuring that resuscitation standards were followed, and not only reflecting on areas in which care is exemplary but also identifying areas that could be improved.

Documentation in the medical record should be concise, legible, and timely. Anecdotal reports and actual record reviews have shown that resuscitation documentation often has not met these criteria. Most nurses can recall recording "code data" on scraps of paper, paper towels, gloves, scrubs, and even bed linens. Entering data into the medical record from these multiple sources is time consuming and difficult after the event. Information recorded in such a fashion often is incomplete because times and details of treatment may be missing, inaccurate, or illegible. If the only available documentation is that recorded after the event, problems with accurate memory of timing, sequence, and performance of events are frequent.

Resuscitation events are often chaotic and result in documentation that may not completely reflect the actions that occurred during resuscitation. For this reason, researchers have attempted to determine what measures will improve resuscitation documentation. This article provides an overview of what is known about resuscitation documentation, discusses the value of using Utstein guidelines [1] in resuscitation documentation, and presents some thoughts for future research related to recording resuscitation events.

Existing comprehensive guidelines provide recommendations to health care providers regarding documentation and reporting of resuscitation events. These guidelines offer recommendations for reporting adult out-of-hospital cardiac arrest [2], reviewing, reporting, and conducting research on in-hospital resuscitation [3], and reporting pediatric advanced life support [4]. Despite these well-developed evidence-based documentation guidelines, there is limited evidence that they are being used as the gold standard for resuscitation documentation.

## Review of the literature

Issues with resuscitation documentation have been present for as long as standardized resuscitation guidelines have been used to guide resuscitation efforts. Researchers and other health care professionals interested in the impact of standardized resuscitation guidelines recognize that essential data elements are not always recorded during a resuscitation event.

### The Utstein guidelines

The Utstein guidelines were developed in 1995 by researchers from the American Heart Association, the European Resuscitation Council, the Heart and

* Cardiovascular Nursing, College of Nursing, University of Kentucky, Lexington, KY 40536-0232.
    *E-mail address:* pkhoward@uky.edu

Stroke Foundation of Canada, the Australian Resuscitation Council, and the Resuscitation Council of Southern Africa to standardize resuscitation definitions and reporting formats [1]. The guidelines are named for the location of the symposium, "Utstein Abbey." These guidelines were based on international expert consensus using scientific evidence to determine best practice for specific clinical situations. The Utstein guidelines recommend that the following elements be documented during every resuscitation attempt: (1) cardiac rhythms, (2) all pharmacologic and nonpharmacologic interventions performed, (3) all event times, and (4) time intervals between interventions.

The Utstein guidelines [1] have provided the most well-known resuscitation documentation template and have made a significant impact on the ability of hospitals to benchmark their resuscitation performance. The success of the out-of-hospital cardiac arrest reporting guidelines [2] prompted development of "Recommended Guidelines for Uniform Reporting of Pediatric Advanced Life Support: The Pediatric Utstein Style" [4]. The adult Utstein Guidelines did not match the needs of pediatric advanced life support, and as a result, a task force was formed to develop pediatric specific definitions. The original charge of this task force was expanded to include data collection related to pediatric resuscitation interventions. The recommended clinical data elements do not specifically reference documentation; however, it would imply that these template variables should be found in the medical record when a resuscitation event has occurred. Other concerns identified by this task force were how to categorize resuscitation efforts in children who are not in cardiopulmonary arrest but are receiving some resuscitation procedures, how to quantify outcomes, and the need for universal pediatric and adult definitions related to resuscitation.

The first paper that recommended application of the Utstein guidelines to in-hospital resuscitation events was published in 1997. These recommendations were designed specifically for documentation of in-hospital resuscitation events and precluded inclusion of events that began on the prehospital environment. The Emergency Cardiovascular Committee of the American Heart Association published these guidelines and developed and disseminated "In-Hospital Resuscitation: A Statement for Health care Professionals from the Advanced Cardiac Life Support, Basic Life Support, Pediatric Resuscitation and Program Administration Subcommittees" [3]. This statement reinforced accurate, timely event documentation using a designated recorder. The report also advocated ethical decision making with regard to

discussion of the appropriateness of (1) "do not attempt resuscitation" orders, (2) use of the American Heart Association "chain of survival," (3) basic life support, early defibrillation, and advanced cardiac life support, (4) quality assurance and improvement for in-hospital resuscitation events, (5) administrative support to allow for ongoing peer review of resuscitation events, and (6) interhospital and intrahospital comparisons of resuscitation events. The Utstein template allows for standardized documentation and is designed to capture time intervals related to resuscitation "gold standards," such as time to intubation [3,5].

*Role of the documentation nurse*

Turjanica [6] describes the role of the documentation nurse as a "key role" during resuscitation events. Emphasis is placed on the importance of good communication between the documentation nurse and the person responsible for overall coordination of the resuscitation event. Responsibilities of the code team documentation nurse are delineated as clarifying, noting time intervals between interventions, accurately noting timing of events, and providing logical transition of events in the medical record, which may include not just the resuscitation form but also the patient's bedside chart or medical record.

*Technology*

Technology was used in an early attempt to improve resuscitation documentation. An electronic clipboard was developed and tested to record events accurately during cardiac arrest [5]. Testing of the device demonstrated no greater accuracy when compared with traditional documentation methods because human factors interfered with accuracy of the device. Although technology has assumed an even greater role in modern practice, an extensive literature search failed to reveal evidence-based information regarding use of automated devices, such as personal digital assistants or pocket personal computers for resuscitation documentation. Anecdotally, it is apparent that computerized technology is being used during resuscitation to guide interventions and record resuscitation events, but clinicians have not formally tested the impact of this technology.

An inability to obtain accurate data from resuscitation events prompted researchers to investigate the use of a barcode system to record accurately the resuscitation event times in a simulated setting [7]. Researchers used the Utstein guidelines [1] as the basis for critical resuscitation event time elements.

Nine subjects watched a videotape that showed a simulated resuscitation. Participants used the bar code device to record each time an event occurred during the simulated resuscitation. Study participants then watched the video a second time and recorded the event times by conventional hand method. The rate of omissions was not different for the two groups. There was a significant difference in the accurate recording of event times ($P = 0.01$), with the bar code group having much greater time accuracy than the conventional method group. This finding is important because the conventional handwritten method should have had greater accuracy based on the second viewing. The repeat viewing of the same video should have had a test-retest effect, which is not what researchers found in this study. The researchers concluded that while human error still had an impact on resuscitation documentation, the use of an automated timing device did improve the recording of times substantially.

*National registry for cardiopulmonary resuscitation*

The National Registry for Cardiopulmonary Resuscitation (NRCPR) [8] was developed by the American Heart Association to serve as a data repository for resuscitation events and allow hospitals to benchmark their resuscitation performance against the Utstein guidelines and that of other facilities. Hospitals may use their own "code sheet" as long as the essential elements of the Utstein guidelines are recorded and can be entered into the NRCPR database. Hospitals that participate in this registry receive quarterly data that depict their performance in the current quarter performance and their performance in the previous three quarters. Eligible resuscitation events for entry into the NRCPR database are those in which a patient experienced respiratory compromise or cardiopulmonary arrest, the facility's personnel performed the resuscitation, and a resuscitation record was completed. NRCPR exclusion criteria include resuscitation events begun outside of the facility (prehospital), newborns in the delivery room, and neonatal intensive care unit patients [9]. Information provided from the NRCPR report assists hospitals in identifying areas that need improvement based on the Utstein standards. The most significant benefit of the NRCPR is the potential to collect data about the care and outcomes associated with in-hospital resuscitation. A limitation of this registry is that only in-hospital resuscitations are included. Future plans for NRCPR development include integrating resuscitation events that begin prehospital with the in-hospital resuscitation benchmarking data.

Participation in the NRCPR program has definite advantages but may not be realistic for all facilities because of cost or other resource concerns. Adhering to the recommendations of the Utstein guidelines provides an excellent template for documentation.

*Resuscitation teams*

Resuscitation documentation is usually a designated role within formal resuscitation or code teams. Documentation during a code may be more accurate when done by a designated code team member for several reasons. The code team recorder should have familiarity with the forms and documentation expectations. As a code team member, the recorder has knowledge of what resuscitation interventions to expect and the importance of documenting these events.

A study was conducted to evaluate the impact of a hospital-wide resuscitation team on patient outcome [10]. This "before and after" study reviewed 220 patients who required resuscitation in the 2-year period. Group 1 included patients whose resuscitation event occurred before the implementation of a formal code team. Group 2 included patients who underwent resuscitation with a formal code team. Patients who required resuscitation in the time period after the implementation of a formal resuscitation team were more likely to experience a spontaneous return of circulation (group 1 = 30%, group 2 = 58%; $P = 0.0002$). Patients in group 2 were also more likely to survive to discharge (18%) compared with patients in group 1 (6%). Once a formal resuscitation team was put into place, more events were recorded. A member of the code team was designated to assume responsibility for documentation, which resulted in accurate recording and sequencing of events. Documentation was believed to be an essential aspect of this hospital-wide resuscitation team.

Because of concern about the accuracy and detail of recording pediatric clinical care, one group conducted a retrospective chart review of pediatric cardiac arrest documentation to evaluate the quality and completeness of the resuscitation event record [11]. Documentation of event details (eg, time, location, personnel) was variable and was absent altogether in approximately 50% of the cases reviewed ($n = 41$). The researchers acknowledged that documentation at the level of detail required during resuscitation was difficult yet essential. They identified that a delay in recording resuscitation event information could result in lost data and that relying on the memory of the health care professional after a stressful and emotional event could further contribute to lost data.

An analysis of 14,720 cases of in-hospital adult cardiopulmonary resuscitation events was conducted to describe NRCPR and provide a comprehensive Utstein-based characterization of in-hospital adult resuscitation. This study was performed using United States data for the reporting period of January 1, 2000 to June 30, 2002 [12]. The analysis provided information about the reasons patients in this registry required resuscitation. The three most common causes of in-hospital cardiac arrest were cardiac arrhythmia, acute respiratory insufficiency, and hypotension. Overall, the subjects had a 44% return of spontaneous circulation, with 17% surviving to discharge. Although this study did not specifically reference documentation, it is assumed that the essential elements as described in the in-hospital Utstein statement [3] were present as the NRCPR database was developed using the in-hospital Utstein statement characteristics.

The review of the literature highlights the lack of critical analyses of in-hospital resuscitation documentation. It is well recognized that documentation during resuscitation is challenging. Many approaches have been tried to improve the accuracy and completeness of medical record entries made during resuscitation. To date, no one method has been shown to be superior, and additional investigation is needed to ensure that resuscitation documentation guidelines are developed scientifically.

*Summary*

Review of the literature found a limited number of evidence-based sources that described what should be included in documentation of resuscitation events. Most health care facilities have established expectations related to documentation of such events based on the recommendations of internal teams that are also usually accountable for developing the "code form" that is used during a resuscitation event. The evolution of the Utstein guidelines has shown that inclusion of specific variables in documentation of the resuscitation event facilitates benchmarking and highlights opportunities for code team performance. The role of technology in resuscitation documentation improves accuracy but still requires human performance for absolute completeness.

of these data elements as the minimum data set to be included in resuscitation documentation. These elements include basic demographic variables of age, gender, and location of event and clinical considerations, such as comorbid conditions, advanced life support in place at time of arrest, previous cardiopulmonary arrest, and reason for admission. Other variables that should be documented include time that resuscitation occurred, time to basic life support measures from beginning of resuscitation event, time to defibrillation use from time that resuscitation was initiated, time to definitive airway management, initial rhythm, and patient disposition at the end of the resuscitation event (ie, stayed in their current location, transferred to intensive care unit, expired). The Utstein guidelines provide well-defined, accepted data categories that delineate key variables as part of the gold standard of resuscitation, which include interval from event onset to start of cardiopulmonary resuscitation, interval from event onset to first defibrillation, interval from event onset to advanced airway management, and interval from event onset to first administration of resuscitation medication. Ultimately, resuscitation documentation must meet the inherent tenets of basic documentation. It should be legible, concise, objective, and timely. Essential criteria of location, number of attempts, who completed the task, time the intervention was completed, patient response, and the route, dose, and site for medication administration should be noted for each intervention. Recorders should be familiar with the forms they are using and be particularly attentive to times. One time source should be chosen for recording purposes. It is not uncommon that in the "urgency" of a resuscitation event times are missed (the recorder was unaware of the event intervention occurring) or just not recorded (too many events occurring simultaneously). Documentation limitations result when data are incomplete, illegible, and not timely.

Resuscitation documentation should provide evidence of the patient's clinical course. Every resuscitation record should give the reviewer a visual image of the sequence of what occurred, who was present, and a patient's final status. The person doing the documentation usually works collaboratively with a patient's nurse to complete any internal forms that are required after resuscitation.

**Recommendations for practice**

Existing evidence and widespread acceptance of the Utstein guidelines make a strong case for the use

**Future research**

Many studies have focused on a review of cardiopulmonary resuscitation, resuscitation events, and patient survival from these events, yet few studies mention documentation. Existing studies have not provided a good correlation of survival rates with improved code team performance and adherence to resuscitation standards [13].

Is there a relationship between code team performance, documentation, and patient outcome? It may prove worthwhile to examine the relationship between timely documentation and overall patient outcomes. Are nurses better able to anticipate patient trends when documentation is concurrent? Is there the potential to change patient outcomes through improved documentation?

Will smaller, smarter technology devices change resuscitation documentation? Does the use of hand-held technology facilitate or hinder resuscitation efforts such as documentation? Do video or audio devices used during resuscitation events improve participant performance during resuscitation and documentation?

There are many unanswered questions about the role that resuscitation documentation plays in patient outcome, nurse satisfaction, and workforce efficiency. Despite all of the evidence and potential for future research, it is important to remember that documentation is an essential aspect of clinical care, not just resuscitation, because such attention to detail in a timely fashion is essential.

# References

[1] Cummins R, Chamberlain D, Hazinski M, et al. Recommended guidelines for reviewing, reporting, and conducting research on in-hospital resuscitation: the in-hospital "Utstein style." Circulation 1997;95(8): 2213–39.

[2] Cummins R, Chamberlain D, Abramson N, et al. Recommended guidelines for uniform reporting of data from out-of-hospital cardiac arrest: the Utstein style. A statement for health professionals from a task force of the American Heart Association, the European Resuscitation Council, the Heart and Stroke Foundation of Canada, and the Australian Resuscitation Council. Circulation 1991;84:960–75.

[3] Cummins R, Sanders A, Mancini E, et al. In-hospital resuscitation: a statement for healthcare professionals from the American Heart Association Emergency Cardiac Care Committee and the Advanced Cardiac Life Support Council, Basic Life Support, Pediatric Resuscitation, and Program Administration Subcommittees. Circulation 1997;95(8):2211–2.

[4] Zaritsky A, Nadkarni V, Hazinski M, et al. Recommended guidelines for uniform reporting of pediatric advanced life support: the pediatric Utstein style. American Academy of Pediatrics, American Heart Association and the European Resuscitation Council. Ann Emerg Med 1995;26(4):487–503.

[5] Ornato J, Fennigkoh L, Jaeger C. The electronic clipboard: an automated system for accurately recording events during a cardiac arrest. Ann Emerg Med 1981;10:138–41.

[6] Turjanica M. Anatomy of a code. Nursing 98 1998; 28(1):34–9.

[7] Stewart J, Short F. Time accuracy of a barcode system for recording resuscitation events: laboratory trials. Resuscitation 1999;42:235–40.

[8] American Heart Association. Making every resuscitation mean more. Currents 2001;11(4):8–9.

[9] Saver C. NRCPR puts heart into improving patient care. Available at: http://www.nursingspectrum.com/MagazineArticles/article.cfm?AID=3428.

[10] Henderson S, Ballesteros D. Evaluation of a hospital-wide resuscitation team: does it increase survival for in-hospital cardiopulmonary arrest? Resuscitation 2001;48:111–6.

[11] Sanghavi R, Shefler A. The ABCs of recording paediatric cardiac arrests. Resuscitation 2002;55:167–70.

[12] Peberdy M, Kaye W, Ornato J, et al. Cardiopulmonary resuscitation of adults in the hospital: a report of 14720 cardiac arrests from the National Registry of Cardiopulmonary Resuscitation. Resuscitation 2003; 58:298–308.

[13] Winslow E, Beall J, Jacobson A. Code blue: what makes a difference? Am J Nurs 2001;101(1).

ELSEVIER
SAUNDERS

Crit Care Nurs Clin N Am 17 (2005) 45 – 50

CRITICAL CARE
NURSING CLINICS
OF NORTH AMERICA

# Use of Handheld Devices in Critical Care

Pamela P. Taylor, PhD, RN, BC

*Middle Tennessee Medical Center, 400 North Highland Avenue, Murfreesboro, TN 37130, USA*

Your patient has just lost consciousness and has a heart rate of 20. You cannot feel a pulse. The patient is not breathing. Quickly you alert the code blue team and find yourself and the patient surrounded with code team members all jumping into action. Quickly, the patient is evaluated and found to be in ventricular fibrillation. The patient is defibrillated once with no response. The patient is defibrillated again, still with no response. The patient is defibrillated once more and converts to a slow rhythm but has no spontaneous respirations and a palpable blood pressure of 50. The code team leader orders intubation of the patient and then looks at you to give medications because the patient was in your care. Based on the patient's status and cardiac rhythm, you prepare to administer 1 mg of atropine and then prepare a dopamine drip. The code team leader asks for 15 μg/min. You know that the patient weighs 96.9 kg. Your mind is spinning from all the excitement and stress of the code. How do you calculate the right amount of medication? What is the formula? Do you multiply or divide? Everyone is watching you. Your mind goes blank. . .

You answer a call for assistance from another nurse whose patient has just had a respiratory arrest. You quickly get the emergency respiratory kit and alert others for assistance. The patient is intubated successfully after several tries by the respiratory therapist. Bilateral breath sounds are noted with crackles and wheezes. The patient is in sinus tachycardia but continues to be dusky in color. STAT arterial blood gases are drawn, and the results are as follows: pH, 7.31; $pCO_2$, 62; $pO_2$, 74; $HCO_3$, 30. What is the next step? How do you calculate mixed arterial blood gas results to identify the primary problem? If the pH is down, is that alkalotic or acidic? The $HCO_3$ and $PCO_2$ are both up. What does this mean?

A young child is admitted to your unit from the emergency department after a motor vehicle accident. The child has numerous fractures in the lower extremities. Roxinol is ordered for pain, but the patient is allergic to codeine. The pharmacy has sent roxicet. Is this the same drug? The medicine room medication reference book is nowhere to be found and the child is really in pain. What should you do?

Emergencies such as these happen every day in the acute care environment, and they demand that nurses quickly make decisions that can have serious, if not potentially fatal, ramifications. Being prepared to make these decisions is partly the result of experience, but having access to ready resources can provide even the newest nurse with the potential to make critical decisions accurately. Locating a specific reference using texts that may or may not be readily available or up to date can be time consuming when time is of the essence. Using personal text-based pocket-sized references—such as for drugs and treatment algorithms—can be helpful, but they tend to be bulky, rarely fit comfortably in pockets, and tend to fly across the hallway when running to an emergency. Handheld devices, such as personal digital assistants (PDAs), can provide nurses with a plethora of instant patient care resources in the palm of their hand, and they are half the size and weight of many of the "pocket-sized" reference books. The adoption of technology by nurses to improve patient safety and care delivery has been slow, however.

*E-mail address:* Pam.Taylor@mtmc.org

## The underlying issues: patient safety and integrating technology into practice

The National Academy of Sciences Institute of Medicine reported in 2000 that between 44,000 and 98,000 people die in US hospitals as a result of medical mistakes, with more than half being preventable [1]. The huge problem with patient safety within the health care industry has received well-deserved emphasis and subsequent actions undertaken to better safeguard the public. Based on information in this report and other research studies, many safety initiatives have been implemented throughout the United States, including the national patient safety goals established in July 2002, by the Joint Commission on Accreditation of Health care Organizations. Additional goals have and will be added each year to further ensure the safety of patients in various health care settings. The goals currently emphasize patient identification, communication among health care professionals, safe medication administration, and handwashing. Compliance with these patient safety goals is required for continued accreditation of the health care organization by the Joint Commission on Accreditation of Health care Organizations [2].

Although health care professionals agree that patient safety is critical, the steps involved to implement these new standards have been labor intensive and actually can slow patient care delivery when using traditional resources and mechanisms to document patient care delivery. The need to improve and modernize the information systems of the health care industry is not a secret held deep within the industry. On April 27, 2004, in a speech related to health care and information technology, President George W. Bush proclaimed that health care was using a "nineteenth century paperwork system" [3]. Relying on print references and information can be costly and pose a huge safety issue. Yasnoff [4] noted that the traditional health care communication of information may lag for a period of up to 17 years from initial discovery until full implementation because of the outdated health care information systems currently in use. Relying on the traditional "print" documentation results in outdated material even before much of the information is available through publication.

The demand for improved safety, patient care delivery, and communication is of great governmental concern regardless of political affiliation and is near the top of the national agenda. President George W. Bush and Democratic nominee John Kerry have proclaimed the need to update the use of information technology within health care to improve patient safety and access. Bi-partisan legislation that pro-motes integration of information technology to improve health care delivery is being pursued in the House of Representatives and the United States Senate [5]. In a statement released in June 2004, by the Subcommittee on Health of the Committee on Ways and Means, the spokesperson noted, "Greater use of IT in the health care field has the potential to reduce medical errors and improve patient care. Many innovative IT projects are underway in both the public and private sectors. Yet widespread adoption of IT in the health care sector has been anemic" [5]. One reason for this slow adoption may be that the information technology skill level of health care professionals has not been highly developed. President Bush noted in an address, "I suspect 20 years ago people who were in the health care field simply could not envision the use of computers and broadband and the Internet to make the field modern. And our education system has got to reflect that. We've got to make sure we train people in the health care field who understand what they're doing when it comes to computers and information technology" [3]. Substantiating this comment, a current review of medical and nursing curricula across the country via the Internet indicates that information technology with specific application to health care is often a missing component in many nursing programs of study.

## Personal digital assistant history and basics

PDAs are not just for busy business executives who manage appointments or computer enthusiasts who explore the latest technology. The term PDA was first used in the early 1990s by John Sculley, president of Apple Computers [6,7]. "Sculley predicted that PDAs would become ubiquitous tools that would hold telephone numbers, keep your calendar, store notes, plus send and receive data wirelessly" [8]. Although a handheld information management tool has been around since the mid-1980s, it was not until the late 1990s that the handheld computer developed widespread use in various industries [6,7]. The newest PDAs have the ability to retrieve quickly and store large quantities of data, including graphics or pictures, perform math calculations at lightning speeds, provide voice recording for quick reminders, and offer decision support material for problem solving and patient management using the latest information from national clearing houses of information related to best practices, such as the Centers for Disease Control and the National Institute of

Medicine. With a few screen taps or mouse clicks, information can be updated as new information is available. Some of the more expensive devices even offer wireless communication and telephone or fax integration [9]. Flash memory in the form of removable cards, such as memory sticks, secure digital cards, and compact flash cards similar to those used in digital cameras, offers potentially unlimited data storage for the PDA [10].

PDAs offer a different functionality than laptops or traditional personal computers (PCs). Besides fitting easily in a pocket, they can be turned on instantly without the traditional "boot-up" of most computer-based systems. Color or gray scale screens are available, although in the health care environment, color screens are preferable and extend functionality [10]. PDAs can be synchronized with a PC to share data via a cable or desktop cradle. The ability to collect data at the bedside and then synchronize the data with a larger health care system improves productivity and loss of information hurriedly scribbled at the bedside on scraps of paper. PDAs also can use a wireless feature to "beam" information to other compatible PDAs, printers, or systems using an infrared transceiver port. Many of the newer PDAs can use wireless technology to access information from a local or wide area network. As the push for electronic medical record systems continues to receive national emphasis, vendors are also building support for the use of PDAs for data input and retrieval within these complex systems, which allow health care professionals to access key patient information instantly while moving from bedside to bedside.

Several well-known vendors, such as Palm, Sony, Hewlett Packard, Dell, Toshiba, Compaq, and Sharp, provide PDAs using either the Palm or Pocket PC operating systems in price ranges from slightly less than US$100 to more than $500. There are two basic operating systems for PDAs that provide the platform for operation. The Palm operating system emerged as the pioneer operating system in the mid-1990s and in many ways has become a standard for health care professionals. Although not as compatible with Windows-based software, such as Microsoft Word or Excel, many third-party software programs allow for Palm- operating system PDAs to download and interact with these popular programs. The Windows Pocket PC operating system, introduced in 2000 as an enhanced Windows CE operating environment, has been gaining in popularity because its interface is most like the Windows environment with which users are familiar on the PC. Although compatible with Windows-based programs, the availability of health

care software for this operating system is still somewhat limited [9].

## Personal digital assistant resources for practice

Numerous software applications are available for the PDA that can provide a safety net at the point of care. This plethora of software for PDAs is primarily available online, which allows for instant access to the software via download. Software for PDAs is available for most any application or specialty imaginable and offers the user an opportunity to customize personal PDAs to provide information resources for a specific patient population or specialty unit. Programmers currently are working diligently to correct the disparity in developing health care software for both operating environments, and many software applications are available in either the Palm or Pocket PC operating systems.

Software prices vary from free to approximately $100 for personal PDA software, with enterprise-wide software (for use on multiple PDAs within an organization) significantly higher. Most vendors allow a trial period for use of the software to ensure that it is applicable to a particular user. In addition to commercial software vendors, many health care professionals have designed software known as freeware or shareware and share it with the public for free or a small fee. Thousands of HanDBase applets (specific database structures designed for various uses) have been built using the HanDBase software program and are available from DDH software. The medical category contains hundreds of applications that can assist the practicing nurse or physician. These applets do require the base software of HanDBase (approximately $30), and they are available for the Palm and Pocket PC operating systems.

There are several useful resources online to assist in the search for specific health care–related software, and new resources are added each day. A metasearch tool, such as with Dogpile (www.dogpile. com) or Vivisimo (www.vivisimo.com), for "PDA AND health care" or "PDA AND nursing" will yield the most current resources. For nurses, several specific Websites exist that provide the latest information related to PDA use in various nursing settings. The *Journal of Mobile Informatics* (http://www. rnpalm.com/) and the American Association of Critical Care Nurses PDA Center (http://aacn.pdaorder. com/welcome.xml) provide some excellent resources and tips for integrating PDAs into nursing practice. A useful general Web resource for health care–related software is HANDANGO (www.handango.com). In addition to health care software resources, this site also provides software for personal productivity, business, education, reference, travel, tools, and even games. An important feature of this software broker is the user rankings, in which users can share their experiences with the software. Searching these resources reveals many software applications for the Pocket PC and Palm operating systems.

In addition to software applications, publishers currently are offering electronic versions of texts and resources for download to the PDA or some removable memory source, such as a secure digital card. Finding the digital text a success in the compact disc version for the PC, Lippincott and Mosby are just two examples of health care publishers that have begun offering resources for the PDA. Resources such as the "Critical Care Handbook of the Massachusetts General Hospital" and Mosby's "Drug Consult 2005" are examples of texts that are available for use via a PDA flash memory card, which weighs fractions of an ounce versus the standard paper text, which can weigh several pounds. A health care professional easily could carry several electronic resources versus traditional paper texts, which would require several backpacks.

PDA information services can provide breaking news related to almost any aspect of health care delivery. Information services, such as AvantGo (www.avantgo.com), provide software that allows the user to select the news services desired. Each time the PDA is synchronized with a PC with Internet access or via a wireless uplink to the Internet, the latest information is downloaded to the PDA for the user to read upon demand. Services such as Reuters, Medscape Mobile, and Health News Digest can provide the latest information related to health care technology and practices; pdaMD can provide tips for all health care professionals for integrating PDAs into all areas of practice.

The latest generation of resources for health care professionals combines several resources, such as medical references, pharmacologic and treatment algorithms, dosing calculators, and other mathematical calculations, that can be used at the point-of-care. Providing clinical decision suggestions, these knowledge-based tools can provide seamless connections through all of the resources via hyperlinks, and a common index provides quick access during even the most stressful patient care situation. In addition to the immediate point-of-care resource, these tools can be configured to display reminders and trigger automatic alerts for adverse drug events

[10,11]. These programs can be helpful for physicians and nurses who practice in the acute care environment, in which accurate and timely decisions can save a patient's life.

## Integration of personal digital assistants into practice

Until recently, many health care professionals have been somewhat slow in the adoption of information technology, such as PDAs [9]. Whereas many medical schools have integrated the use of PDAs as a required tool for medical students, few nursing schools have integrated this component of information technology within curricula to prepare nurses to access and use digital point-of-care information. The benefits of using handheld technology related to patient safety alone are compelling, however.

Let us return to the introductory scenarios of this article. The process for calculating dosages based on weight becomes a few quick data points to enter, and the medication calculator renders the appropriate dose almost instantly. How long would it take to do the math in one's head or on a scrap of paper? Would it be correct, or would a mathematical error have placed a patient at risk?

The second scenario requires knowledge of arterial blood gas measurements related to the physiologic cause and potential algorithms for correcting the imbalance. Experienced nurses may have mastered this content, but nurses who are new in the critical care environment or who seldom deal with respiratory care patients may need some help to communicate quickly the right information to the physician and respiratory therapist. An acid-base analyzer for a PDA would take the reported laboratory values or symptoms displayed by the patient and categorize the disorder and provide possible algorithms for correcting the imbalance.

In the last scenario, the roxinol and roxicet dilemma is solved easily using a PDA-based drug reference that offers drug calculations, interactions, sound-alike/look-alike alerts, and contraindications. A few screen taps would alert the nurse immediately that the pharmacy had sent the wrong drug, in which case he or she could call the pharmacy for the correct drug. There is no need to rely on a medication text that should be located in the medication room but is seldom there when a child is crying in pain.

These powerful resources are all within a finger's reach and have the potential to impact significantly the safety of patient care delivery. Critical care nurses have led the charge when implementing new technology to better patient care, including the areas of information technology. In the 2004 Health Care Information and Management Systems Society (HIMSS) nursing informatics survey, 25% of the nursing informatics nurses surveyed reported that their clinical background began in critical care [12]. These nurses are at the forefront in developing and implementing information technology for safer patient care delivery in a digital environment.

As a population, however, nurses have not readily adopted new technologies related to information technology that can impact patient safety directly and improve the quality of care. According to a 2003 North American benchmark study by Forrester Research in Cambridge, Massachusetts, only 18% of nurses own a PDA compared with 43% of physicians [9]. The fact that medical schools have begun introducing medical students to the PDA impacts this statistic, as does the lack of nursing education related to the use of PDAs. Additional nursing characteristics, such as lack of basic computer skills, nursing shortage, and the average age of the bedside nurse, all contribute to sluggishness in integrating new computer-based technology into daily patient care.

Rogers' "S Curve of Technology Adopters" identifies the characteristics of five categories of individuals as they approach technology integration: innovators, early adopters, early majority, late majority, and laggards [13]. The S-curve model shows that innovation is first adopted by a few people. Diffusion occurs as more and more individuals are exposed to the new technology and begin putting it into practice as they see success by the innovators and early adopters. Momentum with technology integration grows and diffusion reaches a critical mass that proceeds rapidly through the early and late majorities; finally, it slowly spreads to the laggards [13,14]. In many areas of information technology integration, it seems that health care is on the verge of technology diffusion because integration is virtually exploding across the industry and impacting patient care at every turn.

Although health care lags behind many industries in the integration of handheld devices, such as the PDA, tools for assisting health care delivery are here, and the momentum among physicians and nurses is growing. Evidence is readily available to document the impact of information technology on the safety of patients in the health care setting. The use of PDAs can prevent errors and improve patient safety in the critical care environment, where time, nursing skill, and knowledge often make the difference between a patient's life and death.

**Choosing a personal digital assistant**

Choosing a PDA is not as simple as dropping a hint to a family member that a PDA would be desirable gift. The potential PDA user must determine the use and interactivity that is desired based on any requirements for connectivity in the workplace and must evaluate user characteristics. A few key decisions should be made related to the purchase of a PDA.

1. Screen Clarity. Although the gray scale versions offer a less expensive alternative to PDA use, the ability to see the screen in varying light levels is an important consideration. Color screens are also easier to read with aging and tired eyes, which are frequently found in the health care setting.
2. Software Compatibility. One should ensure that any specifically desired software is compatible with the operating system of the PDA.
3. Memory. A minimum of 16 MB of memory is recommended, but 8 MB are sufficient if the device has the capability of expanding by using some form of flash memory cards.
4. Synchronization and Software Loading. A PC is required to synchronize data and upload software to the PDA. A universal serial bus connection is standard for most current PDAs and may not be available on older PCs. Serial connections to the PC can be used but require the purchase of a specific serial cable.
5. Battery Life. The PDA battery life should be at least as long as a typical workday, but most PDA batteries generally last for several days to weeks, depending on the amount of use and type of battery. Additional points to consider include such facts as color screens, which require more battery use than gray scale screens, and add-on accessories, which pull power from the PDA (eg, modems or full-size keyboards) and drain batteries faster than normal PDA use. Spare batteries or a quick-charge cable can be purchased as an accessory for the PDA.
6. Functionality. Determining whether you slip your PDA in your pocket or clip it to your waistband like a pager will drive the choice of case you need for your PDA. Most PDAs come with some type of case, but accessory cases with many different features and colors are available to adequately protect your PDA based on your use and how you carry it with you [10].

# References

[1] Kohn L, Corrigan J, Donaldson M, editors. To err is human: building a safer health system. Committee on Quality of Health Care in America. Washington (DC): Institute of Medicine; 2000. p. 1.

[2] Joint Commission on Accreditation of Healthcare Organizations. Hospital accreditation standards: 2004. Oakbrook Terrace (IL): Joint Commission Resources; 2004.

[3] Bush GW. President Bush touts benefits of health care information technology at Department of Veterans Affairs Medical Center, Baltimore, Maryland, April 27, 2004. Available at: http://www.whitehouse.gov/news/releases/2004/04/20040427-5.html. Accessed July 5, 2004.

[4] Yasnoff WA. National health information infrastructure: key to the future of healthcare. Presented at the Digital Healthcare Conference. Madison, Wisconsin, June 2004. Available at: http://www.wistechnology.com/DHC%20Presentations/DHC%20Yasnoff.pdf. Accessed July 5, 2004.

[5] Klein M. Healthcare technology: on top of the national agenda. Wisconsin Technology Network. Available at: http://www.wistechnology.com/article.php?id=957. Accessed July 5, 2004.

[6] Bayus BL, Jain S, Rao G. Too little, too early: introduction timing and new product performance in the personal digital assistant industry. J Mark Res 1997; 34(1):50–64.

[7] Chew J. Timeline of key events in the evolution of PDAs. Available at: http://www.thecore.nus.edu/writing/ccwp10/james/pda_evo_timeline.html. Accessed July 5, 2004.

[8] Handango. History of the personal digital assistant. Available at: http://www.handango.com/PDAHistory.jsp?siteId=1. Accessed July 5, 2004.

[9] Featherly K, Van Beusekom M. Medicine on the move: PDAs and tablet PCs make the rounds with doctors and nurses. Available at: http://www.healthcare-informatics.com/issues/2004/02_04/PDAs_Gatefold.pdf. Accessed July 5, 2004.

[10] Rosenbloom M. Medical error reduction and PDAs. Available at: http://int-pediatrics.org/PDF/Volume_18/18-2/69_77_ip1803.pdf. Accessed July 5, 2004.

[11] Van Beusekon M. Reducing medical errors: IT helps secure the patient safety net. Available at: http://www.healthcare-informatics.com/issues/2004/05_04/errors_gatefold.pdf. Accessed July 5, 2004.

[12] Healthcare Information and Management Systems Society (HIMSS). 2004 HIMSS nursing informatics survey report. Available at: http://www.himss.org/content/files/nursing_info_survey2004.pdf. Accessed July 5, 2004.

[13] Rogers EM. Diffusion of innovations. 4th edition. New York: The Free Press; 1995.

[14] Cain M, Mittman R. Diffusion of innovation in health care. California Healthcare Foundation. Available at: http://www.chcf.org/documents/ihealth/DiffusionofInnovation.pdf. Accessed July 5, 2004.

ELSEVIER
SAUNDERS

Crit Care Nurs Clin N Am 17 (2005) 51–58

CRITICAL CARE
NURSING CLINICS
OF NORTH AMERICA

# Recommendations of the International Guidelines 2000 Conference on Cardiopulmonary Resuscitation and Emergency Cardiac Care: An Overview

Tom Rone, BSN, RN, CCRN[a],*, Jenny L. Sauls, DSN, RN, C[b]

[a]Intensive Care Unit, Middle Tennessee Medical Center, 400 North Highland Avenue, Box 51, Murfreesboro, TN 37130, USA
[b]Department of Nursing, Middle Tennessee State University School of Nursing, Box 81, Murfreesboro, TN 37132, USA

Despite significant advances in the treatment of cardiovascular disease, it remains the single most common cause of death in developed nations [1–3]. Sudden death related to cardiac cause is estimated to account for approximately 50% of all deaths from cardiovascular causes, most of which are related to ventricular tachyarrythmias [2,3]. The focus of the international guidelines 2000 for cardiopulmonary resuscitation (CPR) and emergency cardiac care was to create widely accepted international resuscitation guidelines that are based on scientific evidence. The purpose of this article is to highlight the recommendations of the international guidelines 2000 conference on CPR and emergency cardiac care and provide an overview of the changes to the advanced cardiac life support guidelines previously published by the American Heart Association in 1992.

## Evidence-based practice

In an effort to fulfill the 1992 goal of producing the first international guidelines supported by international science, the guidelines 2000 participants used evidence-based criteria to establish changes to emergency cardiac care and advanced cardiac life support recommendations published in 1992. The guidelines in 2000 remained largely intact. Topics that were revised or updated used consensus opinion according

to evidence-based practice. The guidelines were classified into three categories according to quality and level of supporting scientific evidence (Table 1). The "indeterminate" category was added to address recommendations that could not be supported or rejected because of insufficient scientific evidence. An international editorial board reviewed the changes for accuracy and potential impact on safety, cost, effectiveness, and teachability [1].

## Basic life support

In 1960, Moss et al [4] first described the effects of closed chest massage. Closed chest CPR remains the standard for maintaining cerebral and coronary perfusion after a cardiac arrest. There is currently widespread consensus that basic life support must be simplified and focus on the essential skills of CPR. Cummins and Hazinski [5] found that only 15% of lay rescuers could assess a pulse within 10 seconds, and 45% reported no pulse when a pulse was present. For lay rescuers, the 2000 basic life support recommendations state that the signal to begin chest compressions is the absence of signs of circulation (ie, breathing, coughing, or movement).

The 2000 guidelines support compressions only for lay rescuers without barrier protection or persons who are unwilling to provide mouth-to-mouth resuscitation. The guidelines confirm that chest compressions alone are beneficial and preferable to not performing CPR (Class IIa). A Belgian Resuscitation

---

* Corresponding author.
E-mail address: thomas.rone@mtmc.org (T. Rone).

Table 1
Classification of therapeutic interventions in cardiopulomonary resuscitation and emergency cardiac care

| Recommendation class | Consensus review by experts |
| --- | --- |
| Class I | Excellent: definitely recommended and supported by excellent evidence with proven efficacy and effectiveness |
| Class IIa | Good to very good: acceptable and useful with good to very good evidence that supports usefulness |
| Class IIb | Fair to good: acceptable and useful with fair to good evidence to support usefulness |
| Class III | Unacceptable: no documented benefit, may be harmful |
| Class indeterminate | Preliminary research stage or insufficient evidence to support a final class decision |

Study Group randomized 520 patients to receive chest compressions alone versus chest compressions with mouth-to-mouth resuscitation from bystanders. They found no significant difference in patients' survival outcomes [6]. The standard chest compression rate for adults remains at 100 per minute. The compression-to-ventilation ratio remains at 15:2 until a professional rescuer arrives and can use advanced airway techniques to secure the airway. At that time, a 5:1 compression-to-ventilation ratio, in asynchronous manner, may be implemented.

Lay rescuers no longer are taught management of foreign body airway obstruction for unresponsive adults. The focus is on maintaining ventilation and perfusion through CPR. As the rescuer performs rescue breathing, he or she should observe for a foreign body and remove it, if visible.

**Electrical therapy**

The initial hope for closed-chest CPR was that circulation and oxygenation could maintain viability long enough to bring the defibrillator to the victim's aid [4]. Early defibrillation is critical to survival from cardiac arrest because ventricular fibrillation (VF) is the most common cause of sudden, witnessed cardiac arrest in adult victims [1]. Time from collapse to defibrillation remains the single most important determinant of survival [7]. The 2000 guidelines stress that early defibrillation (within 5 minutes of emergency medical services notification) is critical to survival and improved outcomes [1]. Many adults in VF can survive and remain neurologically intact even if defibrillation is performed as late as 6 to 10 minutes after sudden cardiac arrest, particularly if CPR is provided [8–10]. Ladwig et al [11] found that patients who did not receive defibrillation within 12 minutes of cardiac arrest only had a survival rate of 2% to 5%.

Many emergency medical services are not able to meet the 5-minute response time recommended by the 2000 guidelines. The advanced cardiac life support guidelines strongly recommend increasing the number of automatic external defibrillators in the community setting and training first responders in the use of these devices (Class IIa) [1]. To support this initiative, the American Heart Association has developed a 4-hour training program—Heartsaver automatic external defibrillator—to provide people in the community with training in CPR and training in the use of automatic external defibrillators. The guidelines also recommend that in health care facilities and related outpatient settings and physician offices health care providers be able to deliver a shock within 3 minutes of a cardiac arrest (Class I) [1].

Research and technology allow health care providers to use lower energy settings to terminate VF. New biphasic defibrillators allow for smaller amounts of energy to be used than with the older monophasic defibrillators. With a biphasic defibrillator, the electrical current is delivered as two pulses of energy in a biphasic defibrillation waveform [1,12]. Research has shown that this two-phased waveform lowers the defibrillation threshold of cardiac muscle, which makes it possible to terminate VF with smaller amounts of energy than would be necessary with a monophasic defibrillator [13].

**Airway management for health care providers**

Airway management is a fundamental component of emergency cardiac care and advanced cardiac life support. Indications for tracheal intubation include (1) inability of the rescuer to ventilate the unconscious patient with less invasive methods and (2) absence of protective reflexes (coma or arrest) [1]. Only experienced and trained health care providers should perform tracheal intubation. Inexperienced providers should use only airway management techniques for which they have been trained and are competent to perform.

In the out-of-hospital setting, unrecognized misplacement of the tracheal tube has been reported in as many as 17% of patients [14]. Confirmation of tracheal tube placement should be achieved by primary auscultation over the epigastrum and right and left sides of the chest. A secondary confirmation should be performed with either an end-tidal $CO_2$ detector or esophageal detection device (Class IIa). Once confirmation of tube placement is verified, the tracheal tube should be secured and monitored closely to prevent dislodgement.

Once the airway is secure, continued hyperventilation is considered to be potentially harmful and should be limited to patients with increased intracranial pressure. Ventilation should be regulated at a rate of 12 to 15 breaths per minute, delivering a lower tidal volume of 6 to 7 mL/kg over 2 seconds [15].

## Advanced cardiac life support pharmacology

In 1992 and in 2000, the guidelines have continued to reduce the number of drugs deemed useful in treating cardiac arrest. Drug therapy during cardiac arrest is considered secondary, and the rescuer should place priorities on basic CPR, early defibrillation when indicated, and airway management [1]. Because of the emphasis on evidence-based research and practice, experts have discontinued the use of high-dose epinephrine as a treatment for ventricular tachycardia and VF. Doses larger than 1 mg do not improve survival and have the potential to worsen postresuscitation myocardial function and neurologic outcomes [1]. Bretylium has been removed from the VF algorithm because of the drug's limited availability and significant adverse effects.

The guidelines for management of asystole and pulseless electrical activity did not change from those previously published in 1992. After initiation of CPR and establishing an airway with adequate oxygenation, intravenous access is initiated and a 1 mg bolus dose of epinephrine should be administered. Epinephrine may be repeated every 3 to 5 minutes if no response is seen. Atropine, 1 mg, may be administered every 3 to 5 minutes for up to a total dose of 0.04 mg/kg in asystole. In the case of pulseless electrical activity or asystole, a review of potential causes (Table 2) should be evaluated in conjunction with administration of epinephrine, because chances of survival are improved with identification and treatment of the cause [1].

Confirmation of asystole requires implementation of the flat line protocol, which includes checking the

Table 2
A potential list of causes for pulseless electrical activity and asystole

| The 5 Hs | The 5 Ts |
|---|---|
| Hypovolemia | Tablets (drug overdose, accidents) |
| Hypoxia | Tamponade, cardiac |
| Hydrogen ion acidosis | Tension pneumothorax |
| Hyper- and hypokalemia | Thrombosis, coronary |
| Hypothermia | Thrombosis, pulmonary (embolism) |

gain, verifying in a second lead, and confirming attachment of all leads and cables. The survival rate for patients found in asystole is as low as 1 or 2 people out of 100 patients suffering from cardiac arrest [1]. Consideration of do-not-resuscitate orders, if applicable, and when to stop resuscitation efforts should be a part of an ongoing assessment by the team leader. New guidelines support end-of-life decisions of terminally ill patients in regard to do-not-resuscitate orders or any documentation to indicate a patient's wish to not be resuscitated. Appropriate respect should be shown for the dignity of patients and families at the end of life in discontinuing resuscitation efforts earlier for patients who have no reversible cause that can be identified or after life-sustaining efforts have been implemented for 10 minutes without evidence of success with persistent asystole [1]. Emergency department and critical care unit personnel also should consider thoughtfully the presence of the family or significant other during the arrest situation.

The bradycardia algorithm calls for administration of atropine, 0.5 mg to 1 mg, intravenously every 3 to 5 minutes for up to a total dose of 0.03 mg/kg (mild symptoms) or 0.04 mg/kg (severe) [1]. Transcutaneous pacing is followed by, in order, dopamine, epinephrine, or an isoproterenol infusion at low doses. If clinicians are concerned about the use of atropine in higher level blocks, they should remember that transcutaneous pacing is always appropriate. The use of transcutaneous pacing is a Class I intervention for all symptomatic bradycardias [1].

Vasopressin, or antidiuretic hormone, is an effective vasopressor and can be used as an alternative to epinephrine for the treatment of adult shock refractory VF (Class IIb) [1,16]. A single 40-unit intravenous dose may be administered [1,16]. Should the single dose of vasopressin be deemed ineffective, the guidelines suggest that epinephrine be given 10 minutes after administration of vasopressin.

The current guidelines recommend anti-arrhythmic drug therapy for persistent ventricular tachycardia or VF that is refractory to early defibrillation. Based on the evidence, amiodarone is currently preferred over lidocaine or procanimide in the treatment of VF or pulseless ventricular tachycardia that does not respond to electrical therapy [1,17]. Amiodarone is an anti-arrhythmic agent that inhibits adrenergic stimulation, prolongs the action potential, and decreases the speed of atrioventricular conduction [1,18]. Amiodarone has been shown to be more effective than lidocaine in the treatment of shock-resistant VF. The Amiodarone for Resuscitation of Out-of-Hospital Cardiac Arrest (ARREST) trial compared 504 patients who suffered out-of-hospital arrest. Subjects were randomly assigned to receive amiodarone, 300 mg intravenously, or placebo before receiving any other anti-arrhythmic drug. The rate of survival for the amiodarone group was 29% higher than the placebo group [17]. The Amiodarone Versus Lidocaine in Pre-hospital Refractory Ventricular Fibrillation Evaluation (ALIVE) trial used a prospective, randomized, double-blind, placebo-controlled clinical trial to compare outcomes of survival to hospital of patients who received lidocaine or amiodarone in refractory VF. In 347 patients with persistent or recurrent VF, 23% of the patients in the amiodarone group survived to hospital admission compared with 12% in the lidocaine group ($P = 0.09$) [19].

In cardiac arrest situations, the recommended dose for amiodarone is 300 mg intravenous push (recommended dilution in 20–30 mL D5W). An additional 150 mg may be given by intravenous push in 3 to 5 minutes, if necessary. The total cumulative dose should not exceed 2.2 g in a 24-hour period. Amiodarone may produce vasodilation and hypotension. It may prolong the QT interval on the electrocardiogram; therefore, administration with other drugs that have similar effects is not recommended. The terminal elimination (half-life) of amiodarone is long and may last up to 40 days [1,18]. In the treatment of wide-complex tachycardia (stable), amiodarone may be administered as a continuous infusion. A maintenance infusion may be used and infused as 540 mg intravenously over 18 hours (0.5 mg/min) [1,18]. Because the solution can crystallize, one should mix infusions planned for administration over 2 hours or longer in glass or polyolefin bottles [1,18].

If hypomagnesemia (serum magnesium level less than 2 mEq/L) is suspected as a potential cause for the arrhythmia or patients who present with torsade de pointes, magnesium is a Class IIb intervention and may be given intravenously in doses of 1 to 2 g. Rapid intravenous doses of magnesium may induce flushing or a sudden sensation of heat. One should use magnesium cautiously in patients with impaired renal function [1,18].

The tachycardia algorithm is divided into four diagnostic categories: (1) atrial fibrillation/flutter, (2) narrow-complex tachycardias, (3) wide-complex tachycardias of unknown type, and (4) stable monomorphic and polymorphic tachycardia [1]. The health care provider must be well trained in arrhythmia recognition to negotiate this algorithm. An assessment also must be made to determine if the patient is "stable" or "unstable." Unstable patients, according to the 2000 guidelines, include individuals who suffer acute ischemia, decreased or altered mental status, heart failure, or hypotension related to a rapid ventricular response [1]. The 2000 guidelines recommend sedation and synchronized cardioversion for patients who have rate-related signs and symptoms that occur with heart rates greater than 150 beats per minute, whereas stable patients are generally treated with pharmacologic interventions.

In patients who present with atrial fibrillation, the 2000 guidelines recommend assessment for the onset or duration of the arrhythmia. For patients in whom atrial fibrillation is present for periods longer than 48 hours, anticoagulation before cardioversion is recommended because of the potential for embolic complications [1]. Calcium channel blockers or beta-blockers are considered appropriate for these patients (Class I). Patients who present with atrial fibrillation of less than 48 hours are candidates for immediate cardioversion (Class I) and are a low risk for emboli.

In narrow-complex, stable supraventricular tachycardias, the guidelines recommend a diagnostic 12-lead electrocardiogram followed by vagal maneuvers and adenosine in an effort to obtain a diagnosis to guide additional pharmacologic interventions. Narrow-complex supraventricular tachycardias can be treated with amiodarone, beta-blockers, or calcium channel blockers if cardiac function is preserved [1]. If cardiac function is compromised, the list of pharmacologic agents is narrowed to only amiodarone. Cardioversion is limited to paroxysmal supraventricular tachycardia and an ejection fraction of less than 40% or patients who are experiencing congestive heart failure [1].

Stable wide-complex ventricular tachycardia with a pulse requires assessment of functional cardiac status with progression to cardioversion and amiodarone if the patient is in heart failure [1]. If a patient's cardiac status is satisfactory, cardioversion and anti-arrhythmic medications, such as amiodarone or procanamide, may be implemented. When in doubt, treat wide-complex tachycardias as ventricular in origin and take into consideration clinical assessment. One always should treat the patient and not the monitor.

In cases of stable ventricular tachycardia that is polymorphic in nature, the health care provider must evaluate the electrocardiogram tracing for prolongation of the QT interval. If the QT interval is prolonged, the rhythm disturbance may be torsade de pointes. Therapies for this condition include (1) magnesium, (2) overdrive pacing, (3) isuprel, (4) phenytoin, and (5) lidocaine. All of these interventions are considered class indeterminate. Medications used to treat monomorphic stable ventricular tachycardia with normal cardiac function include procanamide and sotalol (Class IIa) and amiodarone and lidocaine (Class IIb). In patients with impaired cardiac function, amiodarone and lidocaine are indicated followed by synchronized cardioversion if there is no response to drug therapy. The 2000 guidelines encourage the use of only one anti-arrhythmic agent to avoid synergistic effects and reduce potential adverse side effects [1].

## Management of acute coronary syndromes

Evidence-based data for the management of acute myocardial infarction (MI) has evolved dramatically in the past decade. The primary goals of therapy in management of patients with acute coronary syndromes include (1) reduction of myocardial necrosis in patients with ongoing infarction, (2) prevention of major adverse cardiac events (ie, death, nonfatal MI, urgent revascularization), and (3) rapid defibrillation when VF occurs [1]. Early management of patients who present with symptoms of acute coronary syndrome is critical to salvage myocardial tissue and preserve cardiac function [1].

Initial assessment should include a targeted history and a 12-lead electrocardiogram so that the physician can establish the need for fibrinolytic agents if indicated. If a patient meets fibrinolytic criteria, ideally the fibrinolytic should reach the patient within 30 minutes of arrival at the emergency department. The greatest benefit of fibrinolytic agents is realized if administered within the first 3 hours after the onset of symptoms, yet benefits are still present if given within the 12-hour window recommended in the 2000 guidelines [1]. Depending on local resources, coronary angioplasty is considered the "gold standard" in ST segment elevated MI, because 90% of patients who underwent angioplasty showed improved flow and lower rates of reocclusion than with fibrinolytic therapy [20,21]. All patients who are evaluated and determined to be

experiencing an acute MI should receive initial treatment of morphine, oxygen, nitroglycerin, and aspirin (memory aid "MONA") (Box 1) [1]. Additional pharmacologic interventions should include use of beta-blockers and angiotensin-converting enzyme inhibitors (after 6 hours or when stable), which have been shown to reduce the size of infarction and improve survival of patients who do not receive fibrinolytic therapy.

In patients who present with non–ST segment elevated MI or high-risk unstable angina, the use of aspirin with its antiplatelet properties along with drugs such as reduced dose unfractionated heparin and glycoprotein IIb/IIIa platelet aggregation inhibitors has been found to be beneficial in reducing platelet aggregation and clot formation (Class IIa).

Clopidogrel should be given to high-risk patients with non–ST segment elevated MI if an in-hospital conservative approach is planned or catheterization and percutaneous coronary intervention (PCI) are planned and the risk of bleeding is not high. It is also recommended for patients who have undergone catheterization with PCI and as antiplatelet therapy. The recommended dose is 300 mg by mouth, followed by 75 mg daily for 1 to 9 months. It is not recommended for patients with active pathologic bleeding or patients who have undergone coronary artery bypass graft within the last 7 days. Caution is indicated in patients who have underlying hepatic or renal impairment [22].

Heparin therapy and its use in acute MI is listed as a Class I intervention in patients who undergo percutaneous angioplasty and a Class II intervention in patients who receive selective fibrinolytic agents, such as alteplase, retaplase, and tenectaplase. According to the American College of Cardiology and the American Heart Association 1999 guidelines for management of MI, the dosage for heparin has been reduced to a bolus dose of 60 U/kg followed by an infusion at a rate of 12 U/kg/h (maximum of 4000 U bolus dose and infusion of 1000 U/h in a 70-kg patient). An activated partial thromboplastin time (aPTT) of 50 to 70 seconds is considered therapeutic. The dose reduction of heparin was made to reduce the potential for intracerebral hemorrhage that is associated with higher aPTTs (>70 seconds) [23].

## Management of acute stroke

Stroke is ranked among the top three leading causes of death in most countries and the leading cause of brain injury in adults. The new guidelines place increased emphasis on stroke and afford it the

Angiotensin-converting enzyme inhibitor (especially large anterior wall MI, heart failure without hypotension [systolic blood pressure > 100 mmHg], previous MI)

Patients with ST-segment elevation or presumably new bundle-branch block are candidates for reperfusion therapy.

*From* American Heart Association. Guidelines 2000 for Cardiopulmonary Resuscitation and Emergency Cardiac Care. Dallas (TX): American Heart Association; 2000; with permission.

---

**Box 1. Assessments and treatments to consider for patients who present with acute coronary syndrome**

*Initial assessment*

- Targeted history, including acute myocardial infarction inclusions, fibrinolytic exclusions
- Vital signs and focused physical examination
- 12-lead electrocardiogram; serial electrocardiograms as indicated (postlytic evaluation of ST-segment resolution; recurrent discomfort)
- Chest radiograph (preferably upright)
- Electrocardiographic monitoring

*Initial general treatment (memory aid "MONA")*

- Morphine, 2–4 mg, repeated every 5–10 minutes to provide adequate analgesia
- Oxygen, 4 L/min; continue if arterial saturation is < 90%
- Nitroglycerin, sublingual or spray, followed by intravenous administration for persistent or recurring discomfort
- Aspirin, 160–325 mg (chew and swallow)

*Specific treatments*

- Target times for reperfusion therapy Fibrinolytic agents: door-to-needle time < 30 minutes Primary PCI: door-to-dilation time 90 ± 30 minutes
- Conjunctive therapy (combined with fibrinolytic agents) Aspirin Heparin (especially with fibrin-specific lytics)
- Adjunctive therapy Beta-blocker if no contraindications Intravenous nitroglycerin (for recurrent ischemia, large anterior MI, heart failure, antihypertensive effects)

---

same priority as acute MI. Strokes are classified into two major categories: ischemic and hemorrhagic. Ischemic strokes are associated with an embolic event of a vessel that supplies blood to the brain. Ischemic strokes account for 85% of all strokes combined. Hemorrhagic strokes occur as a result of a rupture of a cerebral artery.

Because reperfusion opportunities exist for stroke patients, time to intervention is crucial for the reversal of ischemia. Intravenous administration of tissue-type plasminogen activator is a Class I intervention and should be administered within 3 hours of stroke symptoms. If administered within 3 to 6 hours of stroke symptoms, it becomes a Class indeterminate intervention. Patients who may be eligible for fibrinolytic therapy must reach a treatment facility and be evaluated quickly to remain within the administration guidelines so that these drugs may be therapeutic and improve outcomes. A patient with a new onset of neurologic deficit warrants emergency room notification and emergency transport to a facility with rapid CT and expertise in the administration of fibrinolytic therapy for acute stroke management [1]. A CT scan is the most important diagnostic tool in differentiating between ischemic or hemorrhagic stroke. Fibrinolytic agents should not be administered until a CT scan has been performed and a differential diagnosis has been made by the physician. Fibrinolytic therapy is not recommended for patients who have a systolic blood pressure greater than 185 mmHg or a diastolic blood pressure of 110 mmHg because of the risk of developing a cerebral bleeding at these pressures. Drug therapy such as sodium nitroprusside, a potent arterial vasodilator, may be used to reduce arterial blood pressure. Antihypertensive therapy may have deleterious effects on cerebral perfusion pressure and should be used with caution.

Emergency medical service systems are encouraged to develop protocols and manage patients with acute stroke in the same manner as they would patients with acute MI or major trauma. Assessment tools have been developed to improve screening in the field and improve recognition of stroke signs and symptoms. The Cincinnati Prehospital Stroke Scale and the Los Angeles Pre-hospital Stroke Screen are assessment tools developed for emergency medical services personnel to screen for acute neurologic deficit in a patient suspected of having a stroke [1]. The Cincinnati Scale states that any evidence of acute facial asymmetry, upper extremity drift, or slurred speech is a sign of a possible stroke. The Los Angeles Pre-hospital Stroke Screen tool addresses neurologic deficit but also includes the victim's age, duration of symptoms, and assessment of other signs that can mimic stroke, such as hypoglycemia and the postictal state after seizure [1].

Key points in the management of stroke are summarized by using the mnemonic of the 7 Ds (detection, dispatch, delivery, door, data, decision, and drug). Detection, dispatch, and delivery are the responsibility of basic life support providers in the community and the local emergency medical services provider. Emergency medical service providers must respond quickly to the call and provide rapid stabilization and transport to the nearest facility that can provide the patient with comprehensive stroke care. After the CT scan, a decision can be made to initiate the final D and treat the patient with fibrinolytic agents [1].

## Summary

Major advances have occurred worldwide in the management of patients with sudden cardiac arrest, acute coronary syndromes, and stroke. In keeping with these advances, the 2000 guidelines for cardiopulmonary care and emergency cardiac care used an evidence-based approach to the development of an international consensus for the provision of emergency cardiac care.

## References

[1] American Heart Association in collaboration with International Liaison Committee on Resuscitation. Guidelines 2000 for cardiopulmonary resuscitation and emergency cardiovascular care: international consensus on science. Circulation 2000;102(8 Suppl): I1–384.

[2] Myerber RJ, Interian Jr A, Mitrani RM, et al. Frequency of sudden cardiac death and profiles of risk. Am J Cardiol 1997;80:10F–9F.

[3] Myerberg RJ, Kessler KM, Castellanos A. Sudden cardiac death: epidemiology, transient risk, and intervention assessment. Ann Intern Med 1993;119: 1187–97.

[4] Moss AJ, Kouwenhoven WB, Jude JR, et al. Closed-chest cardiac massage, 1960. Ann Noninvasive Electrocardiology 2001;6(1):78–80.

[5] Cummins RO, Hazinski MF. Cardiopulmonary resuscitation techniques and instruction: when does evidence justify revision? Ann Emerg Med 1999;43 780–4.

[6] Hallstrom A, Cobb L, Johnson E, et al. Cardiopulmonary resuscitation by chest compression alone or with mouth-to-mouth ventilation. N Engl J Med 2000; 342(21):1546–53.

[7] Cummins RO, Ornato JP, Thies WH, et al. Improving survival from sudden cardiac arrest: the "chain of survival" concept. A statement for health professionals from the Advanced Cardiac Life Support Subcommittee and the Emergency Cardiac Care Committee, American Heart Association. Circulation 1991;83(5): 1832–47.

[8] Eisenburg MS, Cummins RO, Damon S, et al. Survival rates from out-of-hospital cardiac arrest: recommendations for uniform definitions and data to report. Ann Emerg Med 1990;19:1249–59.

[9] Weaver WD, Copass MK, Bufi D, et al. Improved neurologic recovery and survival after early defibrillation. Circulation 1984;69:943–8.

[10] Larsen MP, Eisenburg MS, Cummins RO, et al. Predicting survival from out-of-hospital cardiac arrest: a graphic model. Ann Emerg Med 1993;22:1651–8.

[11] Ladwig KH, Schoefinius A, Danner R, et al. Effects of early defibrillation by ambulance personnel on short and long term outcome of cardiac arrest survival: the Munich experiment. Chest 1997;112(6):1584–91.

[12] Neiman JT. Defibrillation waveforms. Ann Emerg Med 2001;37(1):59.

[13] Jones J, Tovar O. Electrophysiology of ventricular fibrillation and defibrillation. Crit Care Med 2000; 28(Suppl 11):N219.

[14] Katz SH, Falk JL. Misplaced endotracheal tubes by paramedics in an urban emergency medical services system. Acad Emerg Med 1998;5:429.

[15] Melker RL, Banner MJ. Ventilation during CPR: two-rescuer standards reappraised. Ann Emerg Med 1985; 14:397–402.

[16] Linder KH, Dirks B, Strohmeneger HU, et al. Randomized comparison of epinephrine and vasopressin in patients with out of hospital ventricular fibrillation. Lancet 1997;349(9051):535–7.

[17] Kudenchuck PJ, Cobb LA, Copass MK, et al. Amiodarone in out-of-hospital resuscitation after

cardiac arrest from ventricular fibrillation. N Engl J Med 1999;341:871–8.

[18] Lacey CF, Armstrong LL, Goldman MP, et al. Drug information handbook. 10th edition. Hudson (OH): Lexi-Comp; 2002.

[19] Dorian P, Cass D, Schwartz B, et al. Amiodarone as compared with lidocaine for shock-resistant ventricular fibrillation. N Engl J Med 2002;346(12):884–90.

[20] Michels KB, Yusuf S. Does PTCA in acute myocardial infarction affect mortality and reinfarction rates? A quantitative overview (meta-analysis) of the randomized clinical trials. Circulation 1995;91:476–85.

[21] Every NR, Parsons LS, Hlatky M, et al. Myocardial infarction triage and intervention investigators: a comparison of thrombolytic therapy with primary coronary angioplasty for acute myocardial infarction. N Engl J Med 1996;335:1253–60.

[22] Braunwald E, Antman EM, Beasley JW, et al. ACC/ AHA 2002 guideline update for the management of patients with unstable angina and non-ST-segment elevation myocardial infarction: summary article. A report of the American College of Cardiology/American Heart Association Task Force on Practice Guidelines (Committee on Management of Patients with Unstable Angina). Circulation 2002;106:1893–900.

[23] Ryan T. Update: guidelines for the management of patients with acute myocardial infarction. J Am Coll Cardiol 1999;34:890–911.

ELSEVIER
SAUNDERS

CRITICAL CARE
NURSING CLINICS
OF NORTH AMERICA

Crit Care Nurs Clin N Am 17 (2005) 59 – 64

# Update on Pediatric Advanced Life Support Guidelines

Marcia A. Lankster, BSN, RN*, Milton Stanhope Brasfield III, MD

*Bryan W. Whitfield Memorial Hospital, 105 Highway 80 East, PO Box 890, Demopolis, AL 36732, USA*

Accidents are a leading cause of death for children in several nations. Motor vehicle accidents are among the most common causes of cardiac arrest. Other causes include drowning, burns, gunshot wounds, poisoning, smoke inhalation, and airway obstruction caused by asphyxiation from foreign bodies. Approximately 50% to 65% of children who require cardiopulmonary resuscitation (CPR) are younger than 1 year of age, with most being younger than 6 months of age [1]. To prevent loss and improve quality of life, it is imperative to initiate measures to improve oxygenation and treat cardiac dysfunction. Guidelines for the management of life-threatening emergencies in infants and children are internationally similar but not identical. The Australian Resuscitation Council [2], the American Heart Association [3], and the European Resuscitation Council [4] current guidelines all have some basic essential techniques for management of pediatric emergencies.

Children, illness, and injury go hand in hand. When such a medical emergency is more than the parents or guardians can handle, they turn to the medical community. Some of these emergencies inevitably result in a trip to the local hospital emergency department. From the time of the 9-1-1 call to arrival at the hospital and treatment, the health care personnel must possess the ability to manage any and all emergencies.

Immediate and proper assessment and initiation of timely and appropriate medical intervention is vital if the outcome is to be positive. The purpose of life support training is to provide the learner with

the knowledge to sustain basic life functions in the event of sudden arrest. Physicians and nurses in emergency room and critical care settings must possess the ability to act or react to signs of impending emergency. Their timely and thorough implementation of pediatric advanced life support measures are significant factors in determining the ultimate patient outcome.

## Size matters

A child is not a little adult. Treating a child as such can bring about dire consequences. There are basic physiologic differences between adults and children. The need for a specialized area of pediatric emergency management was not recognized during the initial phase of basic cardiac and advanced cardiac life support. Pediatrics was no more than a drug dosage chart in the adult management section of the emergency life support course. To correct this omission, a working group on pediatric resuscitation chaired by Dr. Leon Chaneides was formed in 1978 under the auspices of the American Heart Association Subcommittee on Emergency Cardiac Care. The guidelines for neonatal resuscitation and standards for pediatric basic life support were accepted by the 1979 national conference [5]. The recommendation for a course of study in pediatric advanced life support (PALS) was made by the American Heart Association in 1983. The first manual was complete and a course of study was initiated just 12 years ago in 1988. Revisions were made in 1994 and again in 1997 [6]. Through the years, changes have been made because of technologic advances and good, old-fashioned human smarts.

---

* Corresponding author.

*E-mail address:* mlankster@tha.westal.net
(M.A. Lankster).

## From the outside

Visual changes have been made to the PALS program to enhance the senses of the instructors and participants. The first of these changes can be seen in the actual size of the instruction manual for pediatric life support presented by the American Academy of Pediatrics and the American Heart Association. Going on the "bigger is better" premise, the 2002 edition (2 cm thick) is double the thickness of the 1997 manual. This seems to be more readily attributed to the presentation of the material and not font size or page layout. The original 11 chapters have grown to 17. Additional chapters include information on (1) case scenarios in shock, (2) children with special health care needs, (3) toxicology, (4) rapid sequence intubation, (5) sedation issues for the PALS provider, and (6) coping with death and dying.

For the visual learner, diagrams are dispersed throughout both books. The one-dimensional line drawings on standard paper that appeared in the 1997–1999 edition (Fig. 1) have evolved to full-color, life-like multicultural diagrams on glossy paper in the 2002 manual (Fig. 2). The 2002 PALS manual

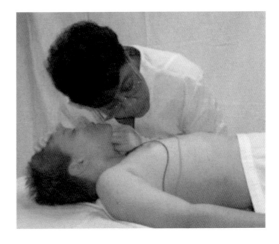

Fig. 2. 2002 PALS manual diagram simulation. Opening the airway with the head tilt–chin lift (as shown for a child). Gently lift the chin with one hand and push down on the forehead with the other hand.

shows the change in the presentation of the material from the typical information and discussion–presentation model to an information and scenario–application model. This format enhances learner comprehension and initiates critical thinking.

## The inner workings

The first procedural change that is evident is the "phone first" versus the "phone fast" approach to emergency medical services activation. The previous routine taught an individual to yell for help and airway, breathing, and circulation assessment in response to finding a person in need of assistance. This was to be done regardless of whether the rescuer was alone. As always, if there are two rescuers, one would activate emergency medical services while the other initiated CPR. Current guidelines allow a lone rescuer to tailor his or her response to the emergency. If the emergency is known, the rescuer should use knowledge of the situation to determine whether to activate emergency medical services or initiate CPR first. If the emergency is unknown, a few guidelines are provided. It is recommended that the age of the victim determine the response. From infancy to 8 years of age, "phone fast" is recommended, with the rescuer initiating CPR first then activating emergency medical services, with the exception of apparent cardiac collapse. For children older than age 8, the "phone first" approach is recommended, with the

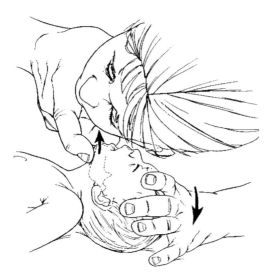

Fig. 1. 1997–1999 PALS manual diagram. Opening the airway with the head lift–chin lift maneuver. One hand is used to tilt the head and extend the neck. The index finger of the rescuer's other hand lifts the mandible outward by lifting on the chin. Head tilt should not be performed if cervical spine injury is suspected. (Reproduced with permission. Pediatric Advanced Life Support. © 197, American Heart Association.)

exception of the child who experiences respiratory compromise or is unresponsive. The 1 minute of intervention before the rescuer leaves the scene is considered beneficial in these victims.

The 1999 guidelines instruct the rescuer in the use of the two to three fingers to the lower one third to one half of the sternum in the performance of chest compressions in an infant younger than 1 year of age. Based on the University of Pittsburgh studies, the American Heart Association has included the two-thumb compression method as an acceptable alternative for infant CPR. Study results demonstrated that the two-thumb method worked better than the two-finger method [7]. This method can be accomplished by the rescuer placing both thumbs on the lower third of the infant's sternum with the fingers wrapped around the infant's back and chest. This method reportedly works better because it combines simultaneous sternal compression with lateral compression.

In the priorities of management, changes have been made in relation to assessment of the physiologic status. Previously, shock was incorporated into the "potential" and "definite" respiratory failure categories. The new PALS guidelines developed a unique and separate category for shock (Table 1). The rescuer is encouraged to look for signs of circulation instead of relying on the presence or absence of a carotid pulse. The rationale for lay rescuers performing a pulse check remains questionable because of its difficulty, and there is strong argument for simplifying the process even further [8,9].

New emphasis is placed on children with special health care needs. The 2000 guidelines define special needs children as children with chronic emotional, physiologic, developmental, or behavioral conditions. When responding to an emergency, although the con-

dition can be the underlying reason for the immediate critical situation, the health care provider should not allow the chronic condition to determine the response. The child must be assessed and emergency medical services activated as recommended.

The lack of medical information, although of particular concern with children who require special health-related needs, is always in the mind of the health care provider. Coupled with the potential for advance directives that would warrant the child not be resuscitated, this information can make the decision to initiate PALS measures one of concern.

Alternative advanced airway devices are addressed in the new guidelines. Endotracheal intubation by prehospital personnel varies by state and expertise of the provider. There has been concern regarding the expertise of prehospital emergency medical care providers in performing endotracheal intubation. In 1983, a 9-month study was conducted in which 178 endotracheal intubations by paramedics were reviewed prospectively. One hundred forty-nine patients (83.7%) had medical conditions and 29 (16.2%) had trauma. One hundred seventy-two (96.6%) of the patients were intubated successfully, whereas 4 patients (2.2%) had unsuccessful attempts made and 2 patients (1.1%) had attempts aborted. There were no reported complications. This study concluded that successful endotracheal intubation could be accomplished outside of the hospital setting [10].

In 2001, the use of endotracheal intubation for airway management in the prehospital setting was revisited in Bobigny, France [11]. Although this study was aimed at adults, it examined the adequate airway management and its outcome in relation to the positive effect on survival or neurologic outcomes. The outcome of this study was controversial. This study indicated the need for improved education of health care providers regarding airway management for out-of-hospital resuscitation.

The requirement for adequate airway maintenance is vital to successful resuscitative measures. With these concerns and the lack of experience and ability to gain necessary experience through practice, the use of endotracheal tube alternatives is becoming more popular. Such devices as the esophageal obturator airway and esophageal tracheal combitube have been used. The laryngeal mask airway, however, is a new device that avoids penetration of either the glottis or the esophageal sphincter, and it provides rapid and easy airway control [12]. It involves blind passage into the airway and is considered simpler to master. It allows a hand-free approach to airway management and can be inserted without the aid of a laryngoscope

Table 1
Cardiopulmonary assessment of physiologic status

| Old guidelines for priorities in management | New guidelines for priorities in management |
|---|---|
| Stable | Stable |
| In potential respiratory failure or shock | Respiratory distress |
| In definite respiratory failure or shock | Respiratory failure: may have increased or inadequate respiratory effort |
| In cardiopulmonary failure | Shock     compensated     decompensated     Cardiopulmonary failure |

or neuromuscular blockade [13]. There are other advantages of laryngeal mask airway: (1) The patient does not need to be supine. (2) The practitioner does not need to be located above and behind the patient's head. (3) Insertion can be done without neck manipulation. A complication to laryngeal mask airway use is severe oropharyngeal trauma, which can result from high cuff inflation pressure. It also does not protect the airway from aspiration of gastric contents in the event of regurgitation. For this reason, it is believed that the laryngeal mask airway should not be used in place of an endotracheal tube during emergency rescue but rather as an adjunct to airway management before intubation [13]. To achieve good outcomes with these devices, the practitioner should maintain knowledge and skills through regular use and frequent practice.

Vascular access is a vital part of the PALS process. Although lipid-soluble resuscitation drugs, such as lidocaine, epinephrine, atropine, or naloxone (mnemonic LEAN), can be administered through the tracheal tube [14], the vascular route is preferable. Once established, intravenous access provides a rapid route for administering critical drugs and fluids with the shortest possible onset of effect. The different needle types and sizes for non-emergent peripheral venous access are denoted in Box 1.

If immediate venous access is not attainable, intraosseous cannulation provides a quick and safe route of medication administration. The 1999 guidelines advocated this route for children aged 6 years or older only if reliable venous access could not be established within three attempts or 90 seconds, whichever came first [15]. The 2000 guidelines no longer dictate this age or time limit. They allow the medical provider to determine a reasonable amount of time depending on the patient's condition. They promote the immediate availability of access as more important than the site of access. The provider is allowed to determine the best site depending on their experience, expertise, and the particular situation.

The cardiac rhythm disturbances of the 1999 guidelines decision trees have become the algorithms of the new guidelines. The algorithms are more detailed and provide guidance and evaluation of condition. Information provided includes not only therapeutic considerations, indications, dose, and precautions but also techniques for medication administration.

The 2000 guidelines discuss nonpharmacologic interventions for treatment of rhythm disturbances. Mechanical vagal maneuvers and pericardiocentesis and electrical defibrillation, synchronized cardioversion, and pacing are presented with consideration of vagal maneuvers added to the algorithm for pediatric

---

**Box 1. Non-emergent peripheral venous access devices**

Newborn, 4–8 kg

- 23- to 25-gauge butterfly needle
- 22-, 24-gauge over-the-needle catheter
- 21-gauge venous catheter needle
- 20-gauge catheter introducer needle

Infant to less than 1 year of age, 5–15 kg

- 23-, 21-, 20-gauge butterfly needle
- 22-, 24-gauge over-the-needle catheter
- 21-, 20-, 18-gauge venous catheter needle
- 20-, 19-gauge catheter introducer needle

One year to less than 8 years of age, 10–30 kg

- 23-, 21-, 20-gauge butterfly needle
- 22-, 24-gauge over-the-needle catheter
- 21-, 20-, 18-gauge venous catheter needle
- 20-, 19-gauge catheter introducer needle

Eight years of age and older, 25–70 kg

- 21-, 20-, 18-gauge butterfly needle
- 16-, 18-, 20-gauge over-the-needle catheter
- 18-, 16-gauge venous catheter needle
- 19-, 18-gauge catheter introducer needle

---

supraventricular tachycardia in infants and children with rapid rhythm. This maneuver can be considered in infants and children with adequate perfusion and only considered in children with poor perfusion if it does not cause a delay in possible cardioversion. It can be attempted while preparing for cardioversion or medication administration.

Automated external defibrillators have been approved for use in children aged 1 to 8 years with no signs of circulation. The PALS Task Force of the International Liaison Committee on Resuscitation made this recommendation in October 2002. There is insufficient evidence for endorsing their use in children younger than 1 year of age. It is recommended that the device deliver a pediatric dose [16]. The task force issued this advisory in relation to automated external defibrillators because of the growing number of adult devices being placed in public settings.

Post-arrest stabilization involves preparation of the patient for transport. PALS currently recommends (1) maintenance of *A*irway patency, (2) maintenance of effective *B*reathing, (3) assessment of *C*irculation, (4) assessment of *D*isability (neurologic function), and (5) monitoring of *E*xposure and *E*nvironment. This adds a "D" and "E" to the standard ABCs of the initiation phase of basic life support.

## International advanced life support

The first European Resuscitation Council guidelines were published in 1992 with collaboration among experts from several European countries [17,18]. The same year, the International Liaison Committee on Resuscitation was formed (with representatives from North America, Europe, Southern Africa, Australia, and Latin America). The aim was to provide a consensus mechanism by which international science relevant to emergency cardiac care could be identified and reviewed. The United Kingdom Resuscitation Council used the advisory statements published by the international liaison committee in 1997 [19].

The basic interventions of cardiac arrest that have proved to improve long-term survival are basic life support and early defibrillation. The most recent and most internationally supported new guidelines are geared toward simplification [20]. The European Resuscitation Council's guidelines match the ideal of describing "appropriate care based on scientific evidence and broad consensus, leaving room for justifiable variations in practice" [21]. These guidelines support the management variability identified in the 2000 PALS guidelines.

## Summary

Management of pediatric patients in emergency departments and prehospital settings represents a challenge for health care providers. The 2000 PALS guidelines provide medical care practitioners with a systematic and organized approach for the management of emergency situations in infants and children. These new guidelines provide nurses and physicians with the knowledge to implement early identifica-

tion and treatment of emergency situations. Up-to-date knowledge of current standards is imperative to promote successful resuscitative outcomes with minimal neurologic dysfunction. Through continued changes and expanded health care provider knowledge, lives of children who experience such emergencies can be saved.

## References

[1] Cardiopulmonary resuscitation. In: Beer M, Berkow R, editors. Merck manual of diagnosis and therapy. 2004. p. 206. Available at: www.merck.com/pubs/mmanual/-33k.

[2] Manual Australian Resuscitation Council. Policy statements: 12.1–12.9. Melbourne: Royal Australasian College of Surgeons; 1995.

[3] Emergency Cardiac Care Committee and Subcommittees of the American Heart Association. Guidelines for cardiopulmonary resuscitation and emergency cardiac care. JAMA 1992;268:2171–302.

[4] Paediatric Life Support Working Party of the European Resuscitation Council. Guidelines for paediatric life support. BMJ 1994;308:1349–55.

[5] Standards and guidelines for cardiopulmonary resuscitation (CPR) and emergency cardiac care (ECC). JAMA 1980;244:453–509. Available at: http://www.uninet.edu/tratado/c1206b.html.

[6] Bardella IJ. Pediatric advanced life support: a review of the AHA recommendations. Am Fam Physician 1999;60:1743–50.

[7] McGaffin M. Two-thumb chest compressions in infant CPR work better than the two-finger method, find University of Pittsburgh researchers. UPMC News Bureau 2000. Available at: http://newsbureau.upmc.com/emergency/InfantCpr.htm.

[8] Eberle B, Dick WF, Schneider T, et al. Checking the carotid pulse check: diagnostic accuracy of first responders in patients with and without a pulse. Resuscitation 1996;33:107–16.

[9] Handley JA, Handley AJ. Four-step CPR: improving skill retention. Resuscitation 1998;36:3–8.

[10] Jacobs LM, Berrizbeitia LD, Bennett B, et al. Endotracheal intubation in the prehospital phase of emergency medical care. JAMA 1983;28(16):2175–7.

[11] Adnet F, Lapostolle F, Ricard-Hibon A, et al. Intubating trauma patients before reaching hospital: revisited. Crit Care 2001;5(6):290–1.

[12] Samarkandi AH, Seraj MA, Dawlatly AE, et al. The role of laryngeal mask airway in cardiopulmonary resuscitation. Resuscitation 1994;28:103–6.

[13] Springer DK, Jahr JS. The laryngeal mask airway: safety, efficacy, and current use. Am J Anesthesiol 1995;22:65–9.

[14] Raehl CL. Endotracheal drug delivery. Pediatr Emerg Care 1992;8:94–7.

[15] American Academy of Pediatrics. Pediatric advanced

life support. Elk Grove Village (IL): American Academy of Pediatrics; 1997.

[16] Samson RA, Berg RA, Bingham R, et al. Use of automated external defibrillators for children: an update. Circulation 2003;107:3250–5.

[17] The Basic Life Support Working Party of the European Resuscitation Council. Guidelines for basic life support. Resuscitation 1992;24:103–10.

[18] The Advanced Life Support Working Party of the European Resuscitation Council. Guidelines for advanced life support. Resuscitation 1992;24:111–21.

[19] Chamberlain DA, Cummins RO. Advisory statements of the International Liaison Committee on Resuscitation (ILCOR). Resuscitation 1997;34:99–100.

[20] Nolan J, Gwinnutt C. 1998 European guidelines on resuscitation. BMJ 1998;316:1844–5.

[21] Thomson R, Lavender M, Madhok R. How to ensure that guidelines are effective. BMJ 1995;311:237–42.

ELSEVIER
SAUNDERS

Crit Care Nurs Clin N Am 17 (2005) 65 – 69

CRITICAL CARE
NURSING CLINICS
OF NORTH AMERICA

# Medication Safety Issues in the Emergency Department

## Margie Brown, RPh

*Bryan W. Whitfield Memorial Hospital, 1310 Forest Brook Drive, Demopolis, AL 36732, USA*

According to the Centers for Disease Control and Prevention, during 2002 an estimated 110.2 million visits were made to hospital emergency departments. During these visits, 75.8% of patients were provided with medication. Because of the urgent nature of these visits, however, most medications are ordered and dispensed without review from a pharmacist [1]. Unfortunately, dosing errors are more common in this setting. Approximately 2000 medication errors occur in the hospital emergency departments annually according to the US Pharmacopoeia, a nongovernmental agency that monitors drug safety [2]. The most common drugs involved in these errors are insulin, morphine, heparin, warfarin, and potassium chloride, which are classified as "high alert" [1].

The Institute for Safe Medication Practices defines high-alert medications as "drugs that bear a heightened risk of causing significant patient harm when they are used in error" [3]. Mistakes may not be more common with these drugs, but the consequences of an error with them are more devastating to patients. The Institute for Safe Medical Practices created a list of potential high-alert medications based on their error-reporting program. Many of these medications are used in the emergency department setting. Box 1 lists some specific high-alert medications [3].

Because of the risk of harm to patients, the Joint Commission on the Accreditation of Healthcare Organizations encourages facilities to handle these medications with caution [4], which is why most facilities no longer store concentrated potassium solutions in patient care areas. They are stored and used only in the pharmacy. The use of prediluted potassium solutions is encouraged to avoid inadvertent use of the concentrated solution.

*E-mail address:* mbrown@tha.westal.net

## Heparin

The high-alert medication heparin is associated with several safety issues. Some look-alike Carpuject products (Abbott Laboratories, Abbott Park, IL) of heparin and ketorolac are commonly used in emergency departments. The syringes have the same green Luer tip cap and similarly colored labels. The company is currently taking steps to improve the labeling of these products. The products both contain bar codes that might prevent an error where technologies exist to distinguish between them [5]. Otherwise, auxiliary labels could be used to bring attention to the name of the drug on the syringe. The dispensing pharmacist should notify all staff who administer medications when a product "look" has changed.

Nurses and medical staff also should be aware that heparin is a weight-based medication. The correct weight of a patient is crucial to accurate dosing of the drug. If asked their weight, some patients may give a false weight because of embarrassment. This misinformation could lead to subpotent or excessive doses when calculations are based on inaccurate weight data. Emergency departments should have policies that promote weighing patients at triage.

A final issue with heparin is concentration. Heparin is available in several different concentrations that range from 100 U/mL (Heplock) to 10,000 U/mL. It is also available in premixed solutions (25,000 U/250 mL). The standardization of floor stock and use of premixed solutions are imperative.

## Insulin

Insulin falls victim to several error pitfalls. There are 23 different brands of insulin, many with confusing, sound-alike names (eg, Humulin 70/30,

| Box 1. High-alert medications |
| --- |

Adrenergic agonists
Adrenergic antagonists
Amiodarone (intravenous)
Cardioplegic solutions
Colchicine injection
Dextrose, 20% or higher
Dialysis solutions
Epidural/intrathecal medications
Heparin, including low molecular
    weight
Glycoprotein IIb/IIIa inhibitors
Lidocaine (intravenous)
Magnesium sulfate injection
Methotrexate
Moderate sedation agents
Nesiritide
Neuromuscular blocking agents
Radiocontrast agents (intravenous)
Thrombolytic and fibrinolytic agents
Total parenteral nutrition solutions

Humalog 75/25, Novolin 70/30, Novolog 70/30). With insulin being associated with the most medication errors in hospitals, safety measures must be implemented in the emergency department [6]. Nurses and medical staff should be educated on all available formulations of insulin used in the facility. Competency testing allows nurses to demonstrate their knowledge about insulin formulations (eg, long-acting versus short-acting) and dosing (eg, common dosing regimens) and helps managers monitor the education level of their nurses and address any education needs.

Nurses also should be familiar with insulin's unit of measure: the unit. The abbreviation for unit— "U"—is often misread as a number, so "5U" may be mistaken for "50." This mistake could lead to dosing errors. For this reason, the abbreviation "U" should be avoided; the word "unit" should be written out on written orders. Preprinted order forms and electronic order entry may help address and offer a potential remedy to the problem with sound-alike insulin names and the misunderstood abbreviation.

Other steps to avoid insulin errors include limiting the floor stock of insulin to regular insulin, standardizing the concentration of all insulin drips, standardizing "sliding scale" orders, and storing insulin in a clearly labeled area of the refrigerator away from any other injectable medications. A standardized list of floor stocks with an established par level also might be helpful.

## Thrombolytic and fibrinolytic agents

Some thrombolytic medications recently have been associated with fatal errors, including tissue plasminogen activator, streptokinase, and alteplase. In a 2000 study at Brigham and Woman's Hospital in Boston, research estimated that 22,500 patients nationally get the wrong dose of clot-dissolving drugs annually, which results in 1500 deaths [7]. Tissue plasminogen activator or activase was associated with the most errors. Thrombolytic therapy for myocardial infarction must begin quickly (within 30 minutes of a patient's arrival to a health care facility). Dose calculation and administration of these drugs are complicated. Situation urgency and a busy emergency department are additional factors that affect accurate medication dispensation. Administration of these drugs requires that a patient receive two separate infusions—a 30-minute infusion followed by a 60-minute infusion. Patients who weigh less than 150 lb also get a lower weight-based dose. Conversely, alteplase (Retavase) was associated with the fewest errors because it is the easiest to administer. Only two injections are required, and they are given 1 hour apart [7]. A new drug since this study, tenecteplase (TNKase) is given as a single injection. It is important that pharmacy and therapeutics committees consider the ease of safe administration when evaluating an emergency department medication. Newer medications may prove easier and safer to administer.

## The Rule of 6

Another error-prone practice in emergency departments that is getting more attention is the "Rule of 6." The Rule of 6 is a method used to calculate concentrations of pediatric solutions in which $6 \times$ weight (kg) equals the amount of drug in milligrams that should be added to a 100-mL solution [8] This practice is riddled with problems. There is room for miscalculations that involve weight conversion in pounds and ounces to kilograms and misplaced decimal points. There are inconsistencies as to where the rule is applied (ie, what drug, what area of the hospital). For example, an emergency department nurse may have to mix a dopamine drip. The nurse uses the Rule of 6 for medication calculation. The pharmacy then receives the order when the patient is admitted. The order is written in milligrams per kilogram per hour. The pharmacist does not know that the nurse already has prepared the solution using the Rule of 6 and enters the order into the computer using a standard premixed concentration (400 mg/ 250 mL). The bag of dopamine would come labeled from the pharmacy based on administration according to the standard premixed concentration. The solution calculation by the nurse and pharmacist would deliver different amounts of drug if administered at the same rate. The nurse who administers the dopamine would have to be cautioned to change the rate on the new bag of dopamine. This occurrence supports the argument that solution concentrations should be standardized whenever possible. The new Joint Commission on the Accreditation of Healthcare Organizations standards and a national patient safety goal require standard concentrations of intravenous solutions [8]. These regulations, in spirit, discourage the use of the Rule of 6. The use of standardized concentrations or premixed solutions throughout a hospital facility would limit the use of the Rule of 6.

## Crash carts

The national patient safety goal that requires standardized concentrations also applies to pediatric crash carts. A standard tool in emergency medicine is the Broselow tape, which can be used in pediatric emergencies [9]. It aids in estimating weight and doses for pediatric medications and the correct size for resuscitation equipment. The tape lists doses by volume instead of weight of drug, which helps to reduce the need for calculations. Use of the tape necessitates the use of the correct concentration of the drug. Atropine, for example, is commercially available in concentrations of 0.1 mg/mL and 0.05 mg/mL. Persons responsible for stocking the pediatric crash cart must be aware of the concentration of the drug listed on the Broselow tape, and it must match what is stocked in the crash cart to administer the appropriate dose of medication [9].

## Nesiritide

The availability of useful cardiac drugs is important to the emergency department. A newer medication used for congestive heart failure is nesiritide (Natrecor) [10]. Approved by the US Food and Drug Administration in 2001, nesiritide is a human recombinant form of brain natriuretic peptide. It is approved for intravenous treatment of patients with acutely decompensated congestive heart failure who have dyspnea at rest or with minimal activity. The first of its kind and the first new agent for the treatment of congestive heart failure in years,

nesiritide is gaining in popularity in emergency departments and intensive care units. Because of the cost of the treatment (average wholesale price US$507.60/vial), the proper mixing and administration of nesiritide is important to avoid waste. The drug is also contraindicated in patients with cardiogenic shock and patients with a systolic blood pressure less than 99 mmHg. The drug dose is weight based. The patient receives a 0.2 μg/kg bolus followed by a 0.01 μg/kg/min infusion [10]. The package insert illustrates precisely how to mix the drug. The 1.5-mg vial is reconstituted with 5 mL of a suitable preservative-free diluent contained in a 250-mL bag of diluent. The resulting solution is then injected back into the 250-mL bag of diluent. The bolus is drawn from the resulting 6 μg/mL solution. The remainder of the bag of mixed diluent is used for the infusion. It is important to label the bag with the exact time and date of reconstitution, because the solution contains no preservative. The solution is only stable for 24 hours [11].

Another issue to consider with this drug is physical incompatibility. It is incompatible with injectable forms of several drugs (Box 2). This information should not mislead physicians, however, because the drugs may be given through another intravenous catheter or after flushing the intravenous catheter. Lasix, for example, is commonly used with natrecor.

Although cardiologists may argue that nesiritide is not a dangerous drug, it is mentioned on the 2003 Institute for Safe Medication Practices' high-alert medications list [12]. Because the dosing is

---

**Box 2. Injectable formulations incompatible in same intravenous line as natrecor**

Heparin *
Enalaprilat
Insulin
Hydralazine
Ethacrynate sodium
Furosemide
Bumetanide
Sodium metabisulfate-preserved drugs

\* Natrecor must not be administered through a heparin-coated catheter. Concomitant heparin infusion must be through a separate catheter. *Data from* ref. [10].

weight based, a dosing chart might be helpful to avoid dose miscalculations.

## Antipsychotic agents

Emergency medicine is faced with many safety issues, some of which have been discussed herein. Even when given properly, some medications produce adverse or undesirable side effects. The resulting side effects may result in repeat visits to the emergency department or admission to the hospital. One such class of medications is the antipsychotic agents [13]. Until recently, acutely psychotic patients who presented to the emergency department were treated with conventional antipsychotic intramuscular formulations, such as haloperidol (Haldol), or benzodiazepines, such as lorazepam (Ativan). These treatments were effective for treating agitation but often produced undesirable side effects. The conventional antipsychotic agents frequently caused movement disorders, such as dystonia, parkinsonism, akathisia, rigidity, and tremor. Catatonia and hypotension were common side effects of these drugs. The benzodiazepines caused drowsiness, behavioral changes, ataxia, and respiratory depression, especially if combined with alcohol or other sedatives [14].

Since the development of atypical antipsychotic medications (eg, clozapine, olanzapine, quetiapine, risperidone, ziprasidone), the use of oral formulations of typical antipsychotic agents (eg, chlorpromazine, haloperidol, thioridazine) has decreased. The limitation of atypicals has been, until recently, the lack of an intramuscular formulation. Currently, two intramuscular formulations—ziprasidone (Geodon) and olanzapine (Zyprexa)—are available. These agents have been found to control agitation and psychotic symptoms rapidly and have a low liability for the adverse effects seen with conventional agents. Because atypical antipsychotic medications have become first-line therapy for schizophrenia and other mental disorders, there should be an improved transition from the intramuscular to the oral formulation. Patient satisfaction and compliance also should improve because of the improved side effect profile. These medications are not without side effects. Some are associated with increased blood sugar levels and prolonged QTc intervals. Although only 3.2% of emergency department visits are for mental health–related conditions, these patients are often a challenge to health care providers [1]. They may be disruptive or violent. The quick and effective treatment of these patients is imperative, which makes these new agents welcome additions to the treatment arsenal.

## Summary

Medication safety and improved patient outcomes are hot topics in modern medicine. Not only are they good ideas in theory but also they are becoming requirements of the industry. The Joint Commission on the Accreditation of Healthcare Organizations has targeted medication errors in its 2005 hospitals' national patient safety goals. One goal calls for the removal of concentrated electrolytes from patient care units. Another goal requires hospitals to standardize and limit the number of drug concentrations available in the facility [15]. Accrediting agencies such as the Joint Commission on the Accreditation of Healthcare Organizations and third party payers such as Medicare are forcing these issues. Practices that are proven to reduce further harm to patients, such as hand washing, taking "time outs" in surgery, and segregating high-alert medications, are requirements and are monitored by accrediting agencies and payors. These are considered not only good practice but also standard procedure. This way of thinking must be performed with new drugs or devices brought into a facility. When introducing a new drug to formulary, not only must the pharmacy and therapeutics com-

---

**Box 3. Safe medication practices for the emergency department**

Standardize and limit the number of concentrations of drugs in emergency department stock

Segregate high-alert medications in the emergency department stock

Avoid the Rule of 6 and use premixed solutions whenever possible

Standardize all crash carts and verify concentrations of drugs on Broselow tape

Limit the number of verbal orders

Avoid using confusing abbreviations (eg, ''U'' for ''unit'')

Separate ''look-alike'' drugs

Conduct periodic competency testing of all staff

Know what drugs are weight based

Post dosing charts for weight-based drugs

Have in-service staff meetings on all new drugs

mittee consider the cost and efficacy of the drug but also it must consider these safety issues. Is the drug dose weight based? What are the contraindications? Where will the drug be stored? Could it be easily confused with another medication? [14] Does the package look like another drug? Is the staff familiar with the drug? Is it compatible with other drugs? These considerations in the early stages of introducing a drug could prove to reduce future errors (Box 3). The safe handling of emergency medications is especially important given the atmosphere in which many are given.

## References

[1] McCraig L, Burt C. National Hospital Ambulatory Medical Care Survey 2002 Emergency Department Survey 2002. Advance Data for Vital and Health Statistics No. 340. US Department of Health and Human Services, Centers for Disease Control and Prevention. Available at: www.cdc.gov/nchs/data/ad/ad326.pdf. Accessed June 28, 2004.

[2] Dobson R. US body reviews errors in emergency departments. BMJ 2003;326:620.

[3] US Pharmacopoeia. Leading medication errors in hospital emergency departments: March 2003. Available at: www.newswise.com/articles/view/?id=EDERRORS. USP. Accessed August 30, 2004.

[4] Joint Commission on Accreditation of Healthcare Organizations. Medication management standard MM.2.20. 2004 comprehensive accreditation manual for hospitals: the official handbook MM-10. Oakbrook Terrace (IL): JCAHO; 2004.

[5] Greenburg L. Carpuject syringe mix ups: medication error report from the institute for safe medication practices. Pharmacy Practice News 2004;31(6):37.

[6] Santell MS, Cousins D. Medication errors: insulin errors, a common problem. US Pharm 2003;28(11): 111–2.

[7] Haney D. Study conducted by researchers at Brigham and Women's Hospital, Boston, MA. Presented at the annual meeting of American College of Cardiology. Anaheim, CA, March 2, 2000.

[8] Grisssinger M. Rule of 6 not optimal for patient safety. Pharmacy and Therapeutics 2003;28(4):234.

[9] Greenburg L. Check your pediatric crash cart: medication error report from the Institute for Safe Medication Practices. Pharmacy Practice News 2004;14.

[10] DiDomenico R, Park H, Southworth M, et al. Guidelines for acute decompensated heart failure treatment. Ann Pharmacother 2004;38:649–60.

[11] Scios. Natrecor dosing information: drug insert. Available at: http://www.natrecor.com/natrecor/dosage. Accessed August 27, 2004.

[12] Institute for Safe Medication Practice. List of high alert medications. Available at: http://www.ismp.org/MSAarticles/highalert.htm. Accessed August 30, 2004.

[13] Hiroto I, Syun Y. Common types of medication errors on long-term psychiatric care units. Int J Qual Health Care 2003;15:207–12.

[14] Brook S. Intramuscular ziprasidone: moving beyond the conventional in the treatment of acute agitation in schizophrenia. J Clin Psychol 2003;64(Suppl 19): 13–8.

[15] Joint Commission on Accreditation of Healthcare Organizations. 2005 hospitals' national patient safety goals. Available at: http://www.jcaho.org/accredited+organizations/patient+safety/05_npsg_hap. Accessed August 30, 2004.

ELSEVIER
SAUNDERS

Crit Care Nurs Clin N Am 17 (2005) 71 – 75

CRITICAL CARE
NURSING CLINICS
OF NORTH AMERICA

# Use of Vasopressors in the Treatment of Cardiac Arrest

## Maria A. Smith, DSN, RN, CCRN

*School of Nursing, Middle Tennessee State University, PO Box 81, Murfreesboro, TN 37132, USA*

Cardiac arrest results from traumatic or medical causes. Victims of blunt or penetrating traumatic cardiac arrest rarely survive this prehospital event. Survival rates vary for individuals who suffer medical cardiac arrest. Internal and external factors affect survival. Internal factors that affect survival include pre-existing conditions, such as ischemic cardiovascular disease and arrhythmias. Out-of-hospital external factors include bystander intervention, emergency medical system response time, and the varied capabilities of emergency units [1]. In-hospital external factors include health care provider capabilities, time to intervention, and patient code status. The goal of resuscitation is to return patients to a physiologic state of wellness that promotes attainment of the best possible quality of life.

It is estimated that cardiopulmonary resuscitation (CPR) is attempted on 370,000 to 750,000 patients annually who have cardiac arrest during hospitalization [2]. Cardiac resuscitation in adults follows a sequential protocol, which consists of rapid access, rapid CPR, rapid defibrillation, and rapid advanced care. These concepts link together to form the "chain of survival" [3]. Quick initiation of these concepts can result in an increased probability for successful CPR.

CPR events result from electrical or mechanical cardiac alterations, such as cardiac tamponade or ventricular fibrillation. Rapid defibrillation is the definitive treatment for ventricular fibrillation and pulseless ventricular tachycardia. The success rate for defibrillation is high when initiated immediately after the onset of the electrical dysfunction, such as ventricular fibrillation [4]. This intervention should be combined effectively with advanced care.

Advanced care includes definitive airway control with endotracheal intubation and pharmacologic therapy. Medication administration is used for arrhythmia management. Cardiac arrhythmias that result in cardiovascular collapse experienced by patients include ventricular fibrillation and pulseless electrical activity (eg, pulseless ventricular tachycardia).

Vasopressors available for use in CPR include epinephrine, norepinephrine, dopamine, dobutamine, and vasopressin [2,5]. The physiologic effects of these drugs depend on adrenergic receptors (adrenoceptor) stimulation. Receptors are classified as alpha ($\alpha$) or beta ($\beta$) adrenoceptors. Both classifications are further divided. Beta adrenoceptor stimulants are subdivided into beta 1 ($\beta$1) and beta 2 ($\beta$2). Alpha adrenoceptor stimulants are subdivided into alpha 1 ($\alpha$1) and alpha 2 ($\alpha$2). These receptors have primary organ locations with varied responses during CPR based on organ stimulation (Fig. 1) [6]. Physiologic response determines indication for use of vasopressors in CPR (Table 1).

Vasopressors are powerful drugs. Intravenous administration results in vasoconstriction and a subsequent increase in blood pressure. The varied ability of vasopressors includes positive inotropic action (increase in cardiac contractility) or positive chronotropic action (increase in heart rate). These actions are critical to successful resuscitation efforts.

## Adrenoceptors

$\alpha$1 receptor activation results in calcium influx across the membrane in certain smooth muscle cells. Pathophysiologically, $\alpha$1 receptor stimulation leads

*E-mail address:* massmith@mtsu.edu

doi:10.1016/j.ccell.2004.09.010

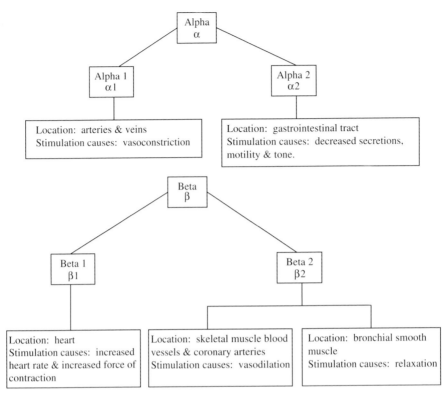

Fig. 1. Primary organ location of adrenoceptors.

to Gq coupling protein. This G protein alpha submit activates phospholipase C. Activation results in the release of inositol 1, 4, 5-triphophate ($IP_3$) and dia-cylglycerol from phosphatidylinositol 4, 5-biphos-phate (Ptdlns 4, 5-$P_2$). Calcium stores are released by $IP_3$ with a resulting increase in cytoplasmic free $Ca^{2+}$ concentration [7]. Various calcium-dependent protein kinases are also activated.

α2 receptors inhibit adenylyl cyclase activity and cause a decrease in intracellular camp levels. Adenylyl cyclase inhibition causes dissociation of the inhibitory G protein by an unclear mechanism. Some α2 receptor effects are independent of their ability to inhibit adenylyl cyclase, including potassium channel activation and calcium channel closure [8].

β1 and β2 subtypes have receptors in various primary organs. Beta receptor activation causes activation of adenylyl cyclase and increased conversion of ATP to cAMP, the major second messenger

Table 1
Vasopressors used in cardiopulmonary resuscitation

| Drug | Receptors stimulated | Indications |
| --- | --- | --- |
| Epinephrine | α1 α2 <br> β1 β2 | Pulseless electrical activity, asystole, ventricular fibrillation, <br> and pulseless ventricular tachycardia unresponsive to defibrillation |
| Norepinephrine | α1 α2 <br> β1 | Acute hypotension and adjunct therapy in cardiac arrest and profound <br> hypotensive episodes |
| Dopamine | α1 β1 <br> Dopaminergic | Secondary shock resulting from cardiac or systemic vascular resistance <br> changes unresponsive to volume infusion, heart block, or symptomatic <br> bradycardia |
| Dobutamine | α1 <br> β1 β2 | Short-term support for cardiac decompensation resulting from depressed <br> contractility states |
| Vasopressin | Vasopressin 1 <br> Vasopressin 2 | Cardiac arrest refractory to epinephrine and defibrillation |

of beta receptor activation. Adenylyl cyclase is the effector enzyme that exerts principal control of cAMP formation [9]. β2 receptor activation promotes smooth muscle relaxation and coronary artery vasodilation. β1 receptor activation increases calcium influx across the cell membrane, where it is sequestered inside the cell [10]. It also causes the release of rennin from the kidney.

Dopamine regulates various functions in the central nervous system and peripheral organs. The effects of dopamine require G couples membrane stimulation and resulting activation or inhibition of intracellular cascades [11]. Dopamine (D1) receptors stimulate adenylyl cyclase and increase cAMP. As a result of cAMP accumulation in the smooth muscle of vascular beds where dopamine is a vasodilator, relaxation occurs. Dopamine (D2) receptors inhibit adenylyl cyclase activity, open potassium channels, and decrease calcium influx. Dopamine (D3) receptors decrease cAMP, open potassium channels, and increase calcium influx [12].

Adrenoceptor response varies. Catecholamines, drugs, patient age, and the presence of diseases may play a role in adrenoceptor number and function on the surface of specific cells. These factors may affect physiologic response to catecholamines. "Desensitization" of adrenoceptors may occur after exposure to catecholamines and sympathomimetic drugs [13]. After exposure of tissue to an agonist for a period of time, that tissue may become less responsive to additional stimulation through drug administration. Clinically, this could affect the therapeutic response of sympathomimetic drugs [14].

# Vasopressors

## Epinephrine

Epinephrine acts on α1, α2, β1, and β2 receptors. Epinephrine is a powerful vasoconstrictor and exerts a positive inotropic and positive chronotropic effect. Effects are dose related. At higher infusion doses, epinephrine exerts a profound alpha effect and is highly vasoconstrictive. At lower doses (0.01– 0.05 μg/kg/min), beta effects predominate. The "standard" resuscitation dose is 1 mg intravenously every 3 to 5 minutes. Research using "high" doses (5 mg) and repeated doses have varying responses [15,16]. β1 adrenoceptor effects increase heart rate and contractile force, which results in increased cardiac output and subsequently systolic blood pressure. β1 adrenoceptor effects also increase myocardial

oxygen consumption and may produce detrimental effects on post-resuscitation myocardial function [17,18]. A reduction in diastolic blood pressure may result from β2 adrenoceptor vasodilation effects in skeletal muscle blood vessels.

## Norepinephrine

Norepinephrine acts on α1, α2, and β1 receptors. The vasoconstriction effects increase systolic and diastolic blood pressures. As a β1 adrenoceptor, it increases heart rate and contractility. This effect is independent of volume. Adverse myocardial effects include ischemia and ventricular tachycardia. An initial dose of 0.5 to 1 μg is given and titrated until the desired blood pressure is achieved. Doses of 8 to 30 μg/min may be required in refractory forms of shock [6].

## Dopamine

Dopamine acts on dopaminergic, α1, and β1 receptors. It is in the central and peripheral nervous system. Dopamine is a neurotransmitter and precursor of epinephrine and norepinephrine. Effects are dose dependent [19]. At doses of more than 20 μg/kg/min, effects mimic those of norepinephrine. At doses that exceed 10 μg/kg/min, α1 adrenoceptor effects predominate, which results in vasoconstriction and an increase in blood pressure. At doses between 2 and 10 μg/kg/min, β1 adrenoceptor effects result in positive inotropic and positive chronotropic effects. Heart rate and myocardial contractility are increased, with a resulting increase in cardiac output. At low doses (1–2 μg/kg/min), dopaminergic receptors cause vasodilation of arteries in the heart, brain, and kidneys [20]. As a result, urine output increases but there is no effect on blood pressure and heart rate.

## Dobutamine

Dobutamine acts on α1, β1, and β2 receptors as a result of a 2-isomer mixture. The α1 adrenoceptor blood pressure response is minimal but may be physiologically measurable in some patients. The selective β1 adrenoceptor agonist effect increases cardiac contractility. Doses range from 2 to 30 μg/kg/ min. At higher doses, chronotropic effects are observed. Doses that exceed 15 μg/kg/min increase the probability of tachycardia and arrhythmias [21]. Although dose related, physiologic effects include increases in blood pressure (especially systolic pressure), heart rate, and vasodilation.

*Vasopressin*

Vasopressin acts on V-1 receptors located on atrial smooth muscle and V-2 receptors located in the renal tubules. The vasopressor effect of this drug is related to action on the V-1 receptors [22]. Vasopressin does not interact with adrenoceptors. For this reason, vasopressin is recommended as a secondary alternative to epinephrine. International cardiopulmonary guidelines recommend vasopressin as a secondary alternative [23,24], although this recommendation is not 100% supported [25,26]. Vasopressin is administered as a single dose of 40 U intravenously. If no clinical response is observed after 10 to 20 minutes, epinephrine, 1 mg, every 3 to 5 minutes can be administered.

**Summary**

Research continues to alter standards of care in an effort to increase survival rate and promote better outcomes for patients who experience CPR episodes. Innovative approaches continue to evolve that incorporate techniques to restore spontaneous circulation and increase survival to hospital discharge. It is important for nurses to remain aware of these approaches and the resulting research. Vasopressors are powerful support drugs in resuscitation efforts that result from cardiac decompensation. To promote the best possible patient outcome, nurses must be knowledgeable of vasopressors used in resuscitation.

**References**

[1] Reichenbach DD, Moss NS, Meyer E. Pathology of the heart in sudden cardiac death. Am J Cardiol 1977; 39:865–72.

[2] Eisenberg MS, Mengert TJ. Cardiac resuscitation. N Engl J Med 2001;344:1304–12.

[3] Cummins RO, Ornato JP, Thies WH, et al. Improving survival from sudden cardiac arrest: the "chain of survival" concept. A statement for health professionals from the Advanced Cardiac Life Support Subcommittee and the Emergency Cardiac Care Committee, American Heart Association. Circulation 1991;83: 1832–47.

[4] Hossack KF, Hartwig R. Cardiac arrest associated with supervised cardiac rehabilitation. Journal of Cardiac Rehabilitation 1982;2:402–8.

[5] Gilmore K. Pharmacology of vasopressors and inotropes: update in anaesthesia. Available at: http://

www.nda.ox.ac.uk/wfsa/html/u10/u1004_01.htm. Accessed July 22, 2004.

[6] Kee VR. Hemodynamic pharmacology of intravenous vasopressors. Crit Care Nurse 2003;23:79–82.

[7] Ruffolo RR, Hieble JP. Adrenoceptor pharmacology: urogenital applications. Eur Urol 1999;36(Suppl 1): 17–22.

[8] Aantaa R, Marjamaki A, Scheinin M. Molecular pharmacology of alpha 2-adrenoceptor subtypes. Ann Med 1995;27:439–49.

[9] Webb JG, Yates PW, Yang Q, et al. Adenylyl cyclase isoforms and signal integration in models of vascular smooth muscle cells. Am J Physiol Heart Circ Physiol 2001;281:H1545–52.

[10] Post SR, Hammond HK, Insel PA. Beta-adrenergic receptors and receptor signaling in heart failure. Annu Rev Pharmacol Toxicol 1999;39:343–60.

[11] Bianche P, Séguélas MH, Parini A, et al. Activation of pro-apoptotic cascade by dopamine in renal epithelial cells is fully dependent on hydrogen peroxide generation by monoamine oxidases. J Am Soc Nephrol 2003;14:855–62.

[12] Missale C, Nash S, Robinson SW, et al. Dopamine receptors: from structure to function. Physiol Rev 1998; 78(1):189–225.

[13] Bünemann K, Lee KB, Pals-Rylaarsdam R, et al. Desensitization of G-protein-couples receptors in the cardiovascular system. Annu Rev Physiol 1999;61(1): 169–92.

[14] Ruffolo RR. Medicinal chemistry of adrenoceptor agonists. Drug Des Discov 1993;9:351–7.

[15] Gueugniaud PY, Mols P, Goldstein P, et al. A comparison of repeated high doses and repeated standard doses of epinephrine for cardiac arrest outside the hospital. N Engl J Med 1998;339:1595–601.

[16] Behringer W, Kittler H, Sterz F, et al. Cumulative epinephrine dose during cardiopulmonary resuscitation and neurologic outcome. Ann Intern Med 1998;129(6): 450–6.

[17] Tang W, Weil MH, Sun S, et al. Epinephrine increases the severity of post resuscitation myocardial dysfunction. Circulation 1995;92:3089–93.

[18] Pellis T, Weil MH, Tang W, et al. Evidence favoring the use of an α2–selective vasopressor agent for cardiopulmonary resuscitation. Circulation 2003;108: 2716–21.

[19] Medsafe. Sterile dopamine concentrate: dopamine hydrochloride. Available at: http://www.medsafe.govt.nz/ Profs/Datasheet/Dopaminehydrochlorideinj.htm. Accessed July 22, 2004.

[20] Bennett WM, Keefe E, Melnyk C, et al. Response of dopamine hydrochloride in the hepatorenal syndrome. Arch Intern Med 1975;135(7):964–71.

[21] Gomersall C. Inotropes and vasopressors. Available at: http://www.aic.cuhk.edu.hk/web8/inotropes.htm. Accessed July 21, 2004.

[22] Goldsmith SR. Vasopressin as vasopressor. Am J Med 1987;82:1213–9.

[23] American Heart Association, in collaboration with the

International Liaison Committee on Resuscitation. Guidelines 2000 for cardiopulmonary resuscitation and emergency care. Part 6: advanced cardiovascular life support. Section 6: pharmacology II. Agents to optimize cardiac output and blood pressure. Circulation 2000;102(8 Suppl I):1129–35.

[24] The American Heart Association in collaboration with the International Committee on Resuscitation (ILCOR). Guidelines 2000 for cardiopulmonary resuscitation and emergency cardiovascular care: an inter-

national consensus on science. Resuscitation 2000;46: 1–447.

[25] Stiell IG, Hébert PC, Wells GA, et al. Vasopressin versus epinephrine for in-hospital cardiac arrest: a randomized controlled trial. Lancet 2001;358: 105–13.

[26] Stiell I, Hébert PC, Wells GA, et al. Evaluation of the myocardial ischemia subgroup in the vasopressin epinephrine cardiac arrest (VECA) trial. Acad Emerg Med 2000;7(5):439.

**ELSEVIER SAUNDERS**

Crit Care Nurs Clin N Am 17 (2005) 77 – 95

CRITICAL CARE
NURSING CLINICS
OF NORTH AMERICA

# Pediatric Cardiac Arrhythmias Resulting in Hemodynamic Compromise

## Vicki L. Zeigler, RN, MSN*

*Texas Woman's University, College of Nursing, P.O. Box 425498 Denton, TX 76204-5498, USA*

Cardiac arrhythmias in the pediatric population share the same underlying mechanisms as those of adults, namely re-entry and automatic/ectopic foci. These mechanisms can result in supraventricular and ventricular arrhythmias. The gamut of pediatric arrhythmias is beyond the scope of this article; however, there are specific arrhythmias that have the potential to result in hemodynamic compromise. These arrhythmias require prompt recognition, rapid clinical assessment, and appropriate clinical interventions from the health care team.

In the pediatric population, cardiac arrest frequently represents the terminal event of progressive shock or respiratory failure rather than sudden collapse secondary to arrhythmias [1]; however, the potential for an arrhythmia to result in hemodynamic compromise always exists. To minimize the risk of cardiac arrest in children with arrhythmias, clinicians must be vigilant in monitoring the arrhythmia to detect early signs of hemodynamic instability. Knowledge of which arrhythmias pose a high risk for deterioration and in whom is critical.

The following discussion is divided into four sections. The first section includes an overview of cardiovascular hemodynamics in children, followed by sections on tachyarrhythmias, bradyarrhythmias, and pulseless arrhythmias. The nomenclature used by the manual on pediatric advanced life support [1] for the latter three sections are fast rhythms, slow rhythms, and collapse rhythms, respectively. Each of the rhythm sections includes a brief over-

view of the specific arrhythmia, electrocardiographic (ECG) characteristics, clinical interventions, and nursing implications.

## Hemodynamics in children

There are numerous anatomic and physiologic differences between children and adults, including— but not limited to—respiratory, cardiovascular, fluid and electrolytes, and thermoregulation. Each can influence a child's overall state of hemodynamics. In pediatric patients, heart and respiratory rates are inherently faster and blood pressure is inherently lower, which make smaller changes in the vitals signs of children more significant than in adults. Critical care nurses who routinely care for neonates, infants, and children are keenly aware that what vital signs are normal for a healthy child (Table 1) may not be what is normal for a child with a structural heart defect.

The primary differences between a child's and an adult's cardiovascular system are faster heart rate and smaller stroke volume. If a child experiences a rapid heart rate (eg, 250 beats/min [bpm]), stroke volume and cardiac output fall because of compromised diastolic filling time and decreased coronary perfusion [1]. Because children have a high oxygen demand per kilogram of body weight as a result of a higher metabolic rate, children depend on heart rate to maintain adequate cardiac output. At the other end of the heart rate spectrum, persistent or profound bradycardia has a similar effect on stroke volume and cardiac output.

---

* 1637 Anchor Way, Azle, TX 76020.
*E-mail address:* vickize@msn.com

0899-5885/05/$ – see front matter © 2005 Elsevier Inc. All rights reserved.
doi:10.1016/j.ccell.2004.09.013

Table 1
Normal vital sign parameters in children

| Age | Respiratory rates* (bpm) | Heart rates (awake)[+] (bpm) | Heart rates (sleeping)[+] (bpm) | Blood pressure (systolic) (mm Hg) | Blood pressure (diastolic) (mm Hg) |
|---|---|---|---|---|---|
| Newborn | 35 | 100–180 | 80–160 | 60–90 | 20–60 |
| Infant | 30–60 | 80–160 | 75–160 | 87–105 | 53–66 |
| Toddler | 24–40 | 80–160 | 60–90 | 95–105 | 53–66 |
| School-age | 18–30 | 65–110 | 50–90 | 97–112 | 57–71 |
| Adolescent | 12–16 | 55–90 | 40–90 | 112–128 | 66–80 |

* Breaths per minute.
[+] Beats per minute.
*Data from* Curley MAQ, Smith JB, Moloney-Harmon PA. Critical care nursing of infants and children. Philadelphia: WB Saunders; 1996.

Respiratory failure in children is characterized by inadequate oxygenation, ventilation, or both. Signs of decreased cardiac output and poor systemic perfusion in children include tachycardia, pallor, cool skin, and decreased urine output. Bradycardia, hypotension, and irregular respirations are late undesirable signs. Because the outcome of cardiac arrest is relatively poor for children, it is crucial that the signs and symptoms of respiratory failure and shock are recognized promptly and that treatment is initiated immediately (Box 1).

To optimize the hemodynamics of a child with a cardiac arrhythmia, any electrolyte disturbances should be corrected. In particular, infants are sensitive to changes in glucose, especially during periods of high stress. Children have higher metabolic rates and greater insensible and evaporative water losses, which results in the need for a larger daily fluid requirement per kilogram of body weight. Because of small absolute fluid requirements, excess fluid administration should be minimized, especially in neonates and infants because of the easy potential for volume overload.

Infants and children have brains that are relatively resistant to hypoxic damage [2]. Critical care nurses and other pediatric health care providers must maintain an awareness of how quickly clinical conditions can change in children and remain vigilant in their clinical assessments. As with all pediatric patients with cardiac rhythm disturbances, continuous monitoring of blood pressure, heart rate, and rhythm is critical. Knowledge of which clinical interventions are appropriate for a specific arrhythmia assists clinicians in caring for children with cardiac rhythm disturbances.

### Tachyarrhythmias

Fast rhythms are by far more common in the pediatric population than slow rhythms or pulseless rhythms. A unique characteristic of children with cardiac arrhythmias is the ability of the body of a child to tolerate these arrhythmias, particularly when compared with their adult counterparts [2]. Tachyarrhythmias in children have the potential to compromise stroke volume and cardiac output as a result of decreased diastolic filling time. The following discussion on tachyarrhythmias in children is not exhaustive but instead focuses on arrhythmias with greater potential to result in hemodynamic compromise. These tachyarrhythmias include supraventricular tachycardia (SVT) in neonates and infants, specifically atrioventricular re-entry tachycardia (AVRT) and atrial flutter, intra-atrial re-entry tachycardia (IART) in patients who have undergone surgery for congenital heart disease (CHD), junctional ectopic tachycardia (JET) in the immediate postoperative period, incessant ventricular tachycardia in young persons, and ventricular tachycardia, specifically torsades de pointes, in patients with the congenital form of long QT syndrome (LQTS).

---

**Box 1. Clinical signs and symptoms of shock and respiratory failure**

Tachycardia
Altered level of consciousness
   (eg, irritability or lethargy)
Oliguria
Hypotonia
Weak central (proximal) pulses
Weak or absent peripheral pulses
Cool extremities
Prolonged capillary refill despite a
   warm ambient temperature

## Supraventricular tachycardia in neonates and infants

SVT is the most common tachyarrhythmia in the pediatric population, with an estimated incidence ranging from 1 in 250 to 1 in 1000 children with structurally normal hearts [3]. SVT is a broad term used to refer to any arrhythmia that originates above the bifurcation of the bundle of His, with rates exceeding 200 bpm in most cases [3]. The most common mechanism of SVT in the pediatric population is re-entry; however, some children may present with automatic/ectopic focus arrhythmias. Some types of SVT seen in children are caused by an accessory connection or AVRT, which may be associated with Wolff Parkinson White (WPW) syndrome, atrial flutter, atrioventricular nodal re-entry tachycardia, the permanent form of junctional reciprocating tachycardia, and atrial ectopic tachycardia.

### Atrioventricular re-entry tachycardia

Approximately 90% of pediatric SVTs are supported by a re-entrant circuit that incorporates the AV node [4]. The term AVRT is used for SVT in which an accessory pathway extrinsic to the AV node completes the re-entry circuit. Concealed and manifest WPW syndromes are the two most common forms of AVRT. The neonatal period is associated with an increased risk of symptomatic SVT episodes, with approximately 50% of children being diagnosed during this period [5]. Many neonates and infants with AVRT present with a 1- to 2-day history of poor feeding, lethargy, irritability, vomiting, or pallor. Although many of these children are clinically stable, within 24 to 48 hours of SVT onset they begin to develop the signs and symptoms of congestive heart failure. In children with concomitant heart disease, congestive heart failure symptoms may appear sooner.

### Electrocardiographic characteristics

The specific ECG characteristics of AVRT can be found in Table 2. In the majority of SVT episodes in neonates and infants, the QRS complex is narrow; however, in the case of existing bundle branch block, the QRS complex will be of the same morphology as that of sinus rhythm. In AVRT, P waves may or may not be visible, but generally are not. The ECG diagnosis of WPW cannot be made until the tachycardia is terminated in most cases (Fig. 1). Neonates can exhibit tachycardia rates ranging from 220-320 bpm [6,7] (Fig. 2) and in 60% of infants with SVT, the heart rate is greater than 230 bpm [8].

### Clinical interventions

In neonates and infants with hemodynamically unstable AVRT, the immediate treatment method of choice is synchronized cardioversion at a dose of 0.5 to 1 J/kg body weight. Cardioversion of AVRT is almost always successful, but if the arrhythmia persists, the dosage should be doubled to 1 to 2 J/kg body weight. This dosage may be repeated once. If multiple attempts are necessary, each shock should be separated by at least 2 minutes in infants and small children to reduce myocardial injury [9]. If intravenous (IV) access is readily available, adenosine may be administered (Table 2), but cardioversion should not be delayed to establish IV access.

In cases of AVRT that are refractory to cardioversion or adenosine administration (ie, the tachycardia is briefly terminated but recurs almost instantly), the anti-arrhythmic agents amiodarone or procainamide can be used (Table 2). Amiodarone has become an increasingly popular anti-arrhythmic agent for hemodynamically unstable tachyarrhythmias in the pediatric age group and has virtually replaced many of the older pharmacologic agents used in the past [10,11]. In the case of AVRT, amiodarone is the pharmacologic agent of choice, but if it is not available, procainamide is second best.

Amiodarone is a potent Class III anti-arrhythmic medication that prolongs refractoriness in most cardiac tissue, which makes it useful for supraventricular and ventricular arrhythmias [12–14]. Because of a multitude of electrophysiologic effects, amiodarone can cause sinus bradycardia, sinus arrest, and AV block. Procainamide is a Class Ia sodium channel blocker that prolongs the QT interval, which makes it prohibitive in patients with acquired or congenital LQTS. It has a known association with hypotension and could result in bradycardia, asystole, depressed ventricular function, or AV block. It should not be given in patients with existing second or third degree AV block without the benefit of a backup pacemaker. Although considered an extreme measure, there are rare cases in which extracorporeal life support has been reported in infants with cardiogenic shock secondary to intractable SVT [15].

### Nursing implications

A child who undergoes cardioversion for AVRT requires continuous ECG monitoring before, during, and after the procedure. It is pivotal that the defibrillator be set to the "sync" mode before energy delivery to deliver a shock that is synchronized to the heart's ventricular activity. Blood pressure monitoring and transcutaneous oxygen saturation monitoring

Table 2
Arrhythmias at a glance

| Arrhythmias | ECG characteristics | Management strategies | Nursing considerations |
| --- | --- | --- | --- |
| AVRT and atrial flutter in neonates and infants | AVRT:<br>Rate: 220–320 bpm<br>Rhythm: regular<br>P wave: absent or negative<br>QRS complex: narrow, unless rate-related BBB or in patients with existing BBB<br>Atrial Flutter:<br>Rate: atrial rate 230–450 bpm<br>Rhythm: regular, if fixed AV block, otherwise irregular.<br>P wave: negative, sawtooth flutter waves (typical) or positive flutter waves (atypical)<br>QRS complex: narrow QRS in most unless BBB present | AVRT and atrial flutter:<br>synchronized cardioversion with 0.5–1 J/kg; if unsuccessful repeat with 1–2 J/kg<br>IV amiodarone<br>Bolus: 5 mg/kg over 20–60 min<br>Infusion: 10–15 mg/kg/d<br>IV procainamide – infants<br>Dose: 7–10 mg/kg over 30–45 min<br>Infusion: 40–50 μg/kg/min | AVRT and atrial flutter:<br>Do not delay cardioversion to obtain vascular access<br>If vascular access available, may administer adenosine at 0.1 mg/kg (100 μg/kg)<br>Do not fluid overload<br>Do not give IV verapamil<br>Use amiodarone with caution in postoperative CHD without pacemaker<br>Monitor serum potassium when administering IV procainimide<br>Monitor serum concentration of procainamide during administration |
| IART in postoperative patients with CHD | Rate: atrial rate 150–300 bpm<br>Rhythm: regular or irregular depending on degree of AV block<br>P wave: small, more discreet, difficult to see; may be hidden in QRS complex or T wave.<br>QRS complex: narrow unless BBB is present | Synchronized cardioversion at 0.5–1 J/kg; if unsuccessful repeat with 1–2 J/kg<br>IV procainamide – older child 15 mg/kg over 30–60 min<br>IV amiodarone 5 mg/kg over 20–60 min | Be prepared for rebound bradycardia or asystole after cardioversion<br>Be prepared to provide temporary pacing<br>Digoxin can be used to slow the ventricular rate<br>Do not place pads/paddles over implanted device |
| JET in the immediate postoperative period | Rate: 110–250 bpm<br>Rhythm: regular<br>P wave: normal, sinus/atrial rate somewhat slower than ventricular rate<br>QRS complex: narrow, unless bundle branch block is present | Induced hypothermia<br>AV sequential (DVI) or AV synchronous (DDD) pacing at a rate slightly faster than atrial rate to provide AV synchrony<br>IV amiodarone 5 mg/kg over 20–60 min | Correct any existing electrolyte abnormalities<br>No direct current cardioversion<br>No overdrive pacing<br>Avoid all catecholamines and sympathomimetics<br>Temporary pacing to provide AV synchrony<br>Keep electrolytes at upper limits of normal |

| Arrhythmia | ECG Characteristics | Treatment | Considerations |
|---|---|---|---|
| Ventricular tachycardia | Rate: Usually more than 120 bpm but at least 10% more than sinus rate<br>Rhythm: Regular in most cases<br>P wave: May be (1) not visible, (2) behind each QRS complex, or (3) completely dissociated from QRS complex<br>QRS complex: Wider than QRS complex in normal sinus rhythm | IV lidocaine 1 mg/kg IVP every 5 minutes for 3 times<br>Lidocaine infusion 20–50 µg/kg/min<br>IV amiodarone 5 mg/kg over 20–60 min<br>IV procainamide older child 15 mg/kg over 30–45 min<br>Esmolol<br>Load @ 500 µg/kg over 1–2 min<br>Maintenance @ 50–200 µg/kg/min | Use largest paddle size possible<br>Esmolol not recommended for long-term use (i.e, >48 hours)<br>Avoid extravasation of esmolol<br>Decrease lidocaine dose with congestive heart failure patients |
| Torsades de pointes | Rate: Rapid<br>Rhythm: irregular<br>P wave: Not visible<br>QRS complex: QRS complexes change from larger to smaller to larger | Defibrillate at 2 J/kg initially, 2–4 J/kg for the second attempt, and 4 J/kg for the third attempt<br>Magnesium sulfate 25–50 mg/kg over 10–20 minutes up to 2 g<br>Lidocaine | Do not give patients with LQTS procainamide or amiodarone<br>Monitor potassium levels (lidocaine more effective with higher potassium levels) |
| Sinus node dysfunction | Rate: Slow for age<br>Rhythm: Regular, unless brady-tachy syndrome<br>P wave: Small and may not be visible if junctional bradycardia<br>QRS complex: Narrow, unless BBB is present | Atropine 0.02–0.04 mg/kg for a minimum dose of 0.1 mg<br>Isoproterenol 0.05 to 1 µg/kg/min<br>Temporary transcutenous pacing<br>Temporary transvenous pacing | Do not give atropine slow IVP because it may cause paradoxic bradycardia in infants<br>Avoid atropine in postoperative brady-tachy patients (enhances AV conduction) |
| Congenital complete AV block | Rate: Atrial rate faster than ventricular rate<br>Rhythm: Regular<br>P wave: Normal but complete AV dissociation<br>QRS complex: Narrow, unless BBB is present | Atropine 0.02–0.04 mg/kg for a minimum dose of 0.1 mg<br>Isoproterenol 0.05 µg/kg/min<br>Temporary transcutenous pacing<br>Temporary transvenous pacing | Do not give atropine slow IVP because it may cause paradoxic bradycardia in infants<br>Assess skin integrity with prolonged transcutaneous pacing<br>Secure temporary pacemaker to patient<br>Assess transvenous catheter site for signs and symptoms of infection<br>Document pacemaker function with ECG rhythm strips |
| Ventricular fibrillation | Rate: None<br>Rhythm: None<br>P wave: Not visible<br>QRS complex: Unidentifiable, variable amplitude, rapid and irregular wave forms | Cardiopulmonary resuscitation<br>Pediatric advanced life support<br>Defibrillate at 2 J/kg initially, 2–4 J/kg for the second attempt, and 4 J/kg for the third attempt | Do not delay defibrillation<br>Continuous CPR<br>Meticulous documentation |

*Abbreviations*: BBB, Bundle Branch Block; CPR, cardiopulmonary resuscitation; IVP, Intravenous Push.

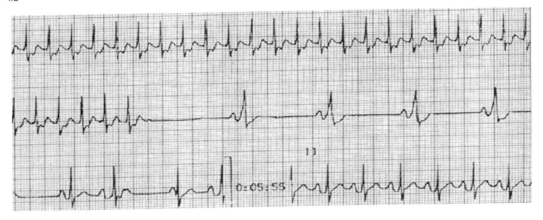

Fig. 1. Continuous ECG rhythm strips of a child who exhibited SVT at a rate of 187 bpm. Adenosine was administered and the first four sinus complexes exhibited the ECG characteristics of Wolff Parkinson White syndrome (short PR interval, wide QRS, and slurred upstroke of the QRS known as a delta wave). The subsequent complexes are completely normal (ie, no WPW, which suggests weak antegrade conduction over the accessory pathway).

should be continuous. If possible, sedation agents should be administered before cardioversion.

Pad or paddle size is important, and the larger, the better. It is important that the pad or paddle have good skin contact. Recommended pad or paddle sizes are 4.5 cm for infants up to 1 year of age or 10 kg and 8 to 13 cm (adult) for children (older than 1 year of age or more than 10 kg) [1]. Pads or paddles should be placed in the anterolateral position or in the ante-

roposterior position in smaller patients or patients with implanted devices.

The child who receives amiodarone should have continuous ECG monitoring, respiratory support, oxygen saturation measurement, and preferably continuous arterial monitoring [9]. Clinicians who care for these patients should be knowledgeable about the intended effects, adverse effects, and interactive effects of amiodarone with other agents. Because

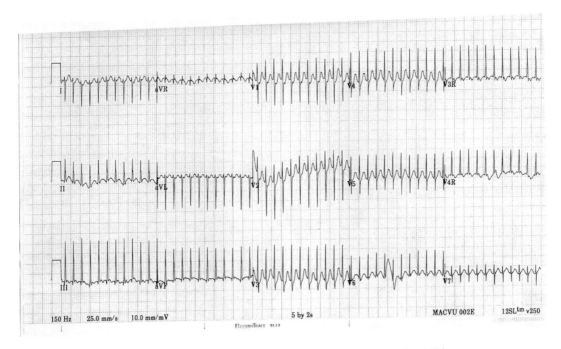

Fig. 2. A 15-lead ECG of an infant with AVRT. The tachycardia rate is fast: 300 bpm.

amiodarone can cause AV block and QT prolongation, frequent assessment of the QT and PR intervals is vital. A 25% to 30% increase in the QT interval may require a reduction in dosage or cessation of the infusion. Transient hypotension, a known adverse effect of amiodarone, can be treated with volume or calcium chloride. It is critical that neonates and infants not be fluid overloaded, so astute monitoring of intake and output is recommended. If a patient is receiving digoxin at the time of amiodarone administration, the dosage of digoxin should be decreased by 33% to 50% to avoid digoxin toxicity [9].

When caring for children who are receiving IV procainamide, the ECG should be continuously monitored for changes in QRS duration, QT interval, and pro-arrhythmia. All ECG changes should be documented with a rhythm strip or 12-lead ECG. The incidence of hypotension in children who receive IV procainamide can be lessened by administering the dose slowly or by using volume expanders. Temporary pacing capabilities should be readily available in the event that AV block occurs secondary to procainamide administration.

Parental education is an important component of caring for children with cardiac arrhythmias. It is critical that nurses take the time to explain to parents the clinical interventions that are being used on their children. Brief, simple, and frequent explanations of their child's clinical condition and the treatment modalities being used will go a long way in reducing anxiety and fear of the unknown in parents of children with cardiac rhythm disorders. Nurses, especially those in emergency departments, who discharge neonates and infants with SVT—or any arrhythmia for that matter—should review the signs and symptoms of tachycardia recurrence with parents or primary caregivers and assist them in devising a plan should the child have a recurrence.

### Atrial flutter

Atrial flutter is uncommon in children with anatomically normal hearts and is limited primarily to infants. Atrial flutter accounts for 30% of fetal tachycardias [16], 18% of neonatal tachyarrhythmias [17], and 8% of SVTs in children older than 1 year of age [18]. This tachyarrhythmia results from a macrore-entrant circuit around fixed or functional barriers, with areas of relatively slow conduction and unidirectional block.

### Electrocardiographic characteristics

The ECG characteristics of atrial flutter can be found in Table 2. Neonates and infants with atrial

flutter can exhibit high atrial (flutter) rates that range from 230 to 450 bpm [5], with slower ventricular rates ranging from 150 to 300 bpm. Although the atrial rate in flutter is important, it is usually the degree of AV block (ie, how many flutter waves are actually conducted to the ventricles) that is responsible for hemodynamic compromise (Fig. 3). In most cases, there is 2:1 or 3:1 AV block, but in rare cases, there is 1:1 AV conduction.

### Clinical interventions

Symptomatic neonates and infants may present with tachypnea, poor feeding, and diaphoresis. The longer a child experiences sustained atrial flutter, the more likely he or she is to develop congestive heart failure. In hemodynamically compromised neonates and infants with atrial flutter, the treatment method of choice is synchronized cardioversion, which almost always terminates the tachycardia. Similar to the treatment of AVRT, amiodarone and procainamide also can be used, but procainamide administration can result in an increased ventricular response when given to patients with atrial flutter. Digoxin can be used to slow the ventricular rate, as can the beta blocker esmolol, which has been used successfully in patients with atrial flutter [9].

Esmolol hydrochloride is a Class II, ultra short-acting beta-adrenergic blocker and should be used only if ventricular function permits because of its negative inotropic effects. It should be avoided in patients with overt heart failure and used with extreme caution if ventricular function is depressed [9]. It may be used to slow the ventricular rate acutely, if necessary, while other treatment options are explored. Other beta blockers should not be used intravenously during esmolol administration. Because of its pro-

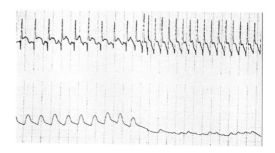

Fig. 3. Simultaneous ECG rhythm strip and arterial blood pressure measurement. In the first half of the recording, the infant exhibited atrial flutter with 2:1 AV block and an adequate blood pressure. In the second half of the recording, the atrial flutter conducted 1:1, which caused an immediate drop in arterial pressure.

pensity to depress ventricular function, a baseline evaluation using echocardiography is recommended.

*Nursing implications*

The nursing implications for neonates and infants with atrial flutter are essentially the same as those for the children who experience AVRT. The nursing implications regarding cardioversion, amiodarone, procainamide, and parental education can be found in the previous section on AVRT.

More than half of patients who receive esmolol exhibit hypotension, especially with bolus administration. The incidence of hypotension is increased in smaller children [19] but can be reduced by administering the agent more slowly in these patients. The effects of esmolol can be reversed with volume, calcium chloride, or a reduction in dosage. Nurses

should monitor continuously the IV site for signs of infiltration, because extravasation can produce skin necrosis.

*Intra-atrial re-entry tachycardia in postoperative patients with congenital heart disease*

Cardiac rhythm disturbances experienced after surgery for CHD can occur because of injury to the conduction system, ischemia, suture placement near the conduction system, altered hemodynamics, electrolyte imbalances, and medications [20]. The term "intra-atrial re-entry tachycardia" (IART) is a diagnostic term used by pediatric cardiovascular health care providers to refer to an atrial re-entrant rhythm in the presence of CHD [5]. In most cases, the surgical

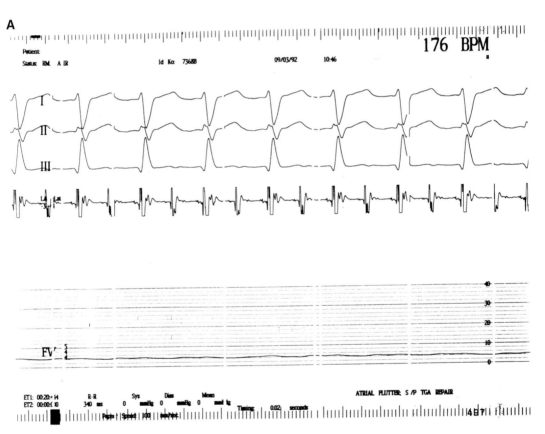

Fig. 4. (*A*) Surface ECG recording of leads I, II, and III in a patient after Mustard repair for d-TGA. The fourth electrogram was recorded from the right atrium showing atrial flutter waves not easily identified from the surface ECG. With 2:1 AV conduction of the flutter, the ventricular rate is fast (176 bpm) for a child with altered cardiac physiology. (*B*) Same patient as in *A*. The flutter continued despite adenosine administration as evidenced by the atrial electrogram, but the medication produced greater AV block, which indicated that the arrhythmia was IART, which does not need the AV node for perpetuation. (*C*) Same patient as in *A* and *B* after synchronized cardioversion. The intracardiac electrogram exhibited normal sinus rhythm with 1:1 AV conduction at 105 bpm.

procedure involved or affected the atrium, primarily the right atrium. The re-entry circuit is within the atrial tissue itself and occurs as a result of scarring or increased intra-atrial pressure. Surgical procedures associated with an increased risk of postoperative IART include atrial septal defect, the Mustard or Senning repair for transposition of the great arteries, and the Fontan procedure [21,22].

*Electrocardiographic characteristics*

Specific ECG characteristics of IART in patients who have previously undergone surgery for CHD can be found in Table 2. This tachyarrhythmia generally results in a slower ventricular rate compared with typical or atypical forms of atrial flutter. In contrast to neonates and infants with atrial flutter, these patients may have small, difficult-to-see flutter waves on the surface ECG without the classic "sawtooth" appearance (Fig. 4A–C) [5]. They may be hidden in the QRS complex or the T wave. The most apparent danger for these patients is a 1:1 conduction of atrial flutter waves.

*Clinical interventions*

After atrial flutter has been confirmed by adenosine administration, which creates additional block without terminating the flutter, the postoperative patient with IART immediately should undergo synchronized cardioversion at a dose of 0.5 to 1 J/kg body weight. In more stable patients, atrial overdrive pacing may be performed. If a child is in the immediate postoperative period, the temporary epicardial pacing wires may be used to overdrive the atrium; however, other patients may require insertion of a temporary pacing electrode by transesophageal or transvenous approach.

In patients with IART, there is a high risk of underlying sinus bradycardia after conversion of the tachyarrhythmia. Digoxin may be used to slow the ventricular rate, but most anti-arrhythmic agents may further compromise sinus node function and should be used with caution. The postoperative state also predisposes these patients to intracardiac thrombi, which may become dislodged by cardioversion and necessitate the use of transesophageal echocardiog-

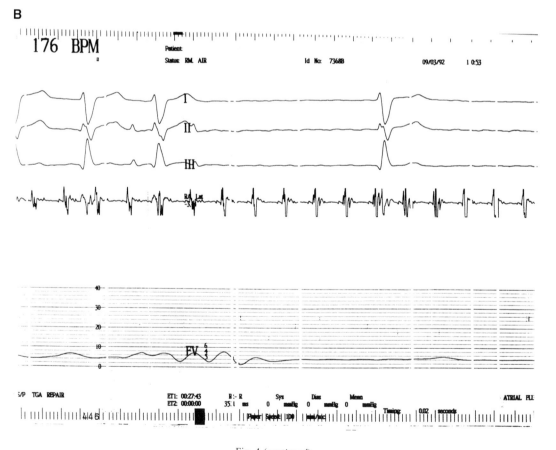

Fig. 4 (*continued*).

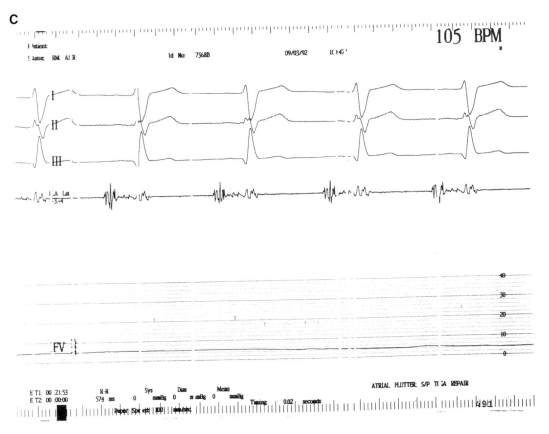

Fig. 4 (*continued*).

raphy at the time of cardioversion. If thrombi are visualized, the patient must be anticoagulated before cardioversion. IV amiodarone is also an option for these patients.

*Nursing implications*

The nursing implications for children with IART are similar to those for SVT in neonates and infants. Because of the propensity for patients with IART to experience rebound bradycardia or asystole after cardioversion, temporary pacing should be readily available. Most modern defibrillators have the ability to provide temporary pacing, and nurses must be familiar with the operation of the pacemaker component before cardioversion. The time to learn how to use this function is not during an episode of bradycardia or asystole after cardioversion. When placing pads or paddles on patients with implanted cardiac devices (ie, pacemakers or defibrillators), care should be taken not to place them over the device. Not only can the device block current flow but also the pad or paddles could impair skin integrity near the device pocket and predispose patients to infection.

Atrial overdrive pacing can be successful in terminating IART. If using the postoperative epicardial pacing wires, gloves should be worn when handling the wires to prevent the inadvertent transfer of static electricity to a patient through the wires. If using a percutaneous or esophageal catheter, the catheter should be secured properly at the exit site. A rate slightly faster than the atrial flutter rate is used to overdrive suppress the atrium to interrupt the re-entry circuit [23]. To disrupt the re-entry circuit, atrial pacing is stopped abruptly.

Parents and primary caregivers should receive information regarding the various clinical interventions used to treat their child's tachyarrhythmia. Because there is a good chance for recurrence of IART in these patients, information regarding long-term treatment options should be made readily available.

*Junctional ectopic tachycardia in the immediate postoperative period*

JET is a form of ectopic (automatic) tachycardia that arises from the bundle of His. It accounts for only

8% of all SVTs in children [24] and can occur after surgery for any defect that involves the right atrium, the right ventricle, or both. It occurs as a result of irritation (eg, edema or suture placement) of the bundle of His during the repair. The initial presentation can be misleading because the junctional/ventricular rate starts out slow but can accelerate quickly in the first 24 to 48 hours after surgery. This acceleration in the ventricular rate rapidly exceeds that of the sinus/atrial rate, which leads to the loss of atrioventricular synchrony (Fig. 5). This loss of AV synchrony in turn leads to hemodynamic instability and compromise because of the subsequent decrease in cardiac output. The arrhythmia is generally self-limiting (48–72 hours) if efforts are undertaken that promote increased vagal tone, decreased adrenergic/sympathetic tone, and increased cardiac output.

*Electrocardiographic characteristics*

The ECG characteristics for JET can be found in Table 2. A multichannel ECG is generally sufficient to make the diagnosis, but occasionally a temporary atrial pacing wire or transesophageal electrode recording is necessary to ascertain the AV relationship. In most cases of JET, there is a narrow QRS complex, unless surgery has resulted in bundle branch block. The QRS morphology of the JET is generally the same QRS morphology as that of sinus rhythm, and the P waves just "march" through the junctional rhythm at a slower rate.

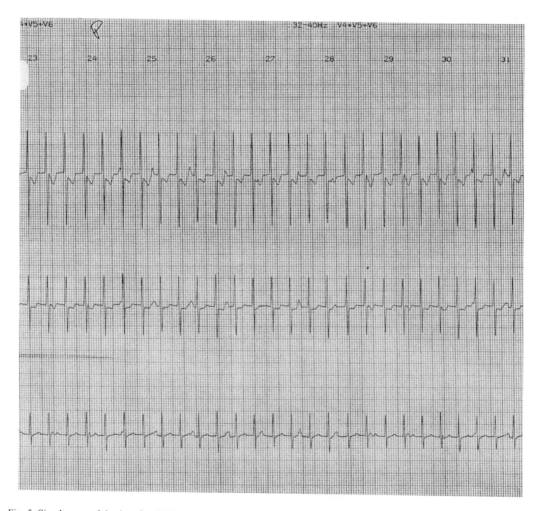

Fig. 5. Simultaneous 3-lead surface ECG recording of a patient who exhibited JET. The QRS complex is normal (narrow) and AV dissociation is evident in all three leads. Many of the P waves (the rate of which is slightly slower than the QRS rate) are buried in the T waves, which give the T waves an irregular morphology.

## Clinical interventions

This transient arrhythmia is likely to resolve in hours or days if supportive measures are undertaken quickly to improve hemodynamics. One of the problems with this arrhythmia is that it does not respond to interventions that are commonly used to terminate re-entrant arrhythmias, such as cardioversion or overdrive pacing. It is also refractory to most anti-arrhythmic drugs. The treatment goals of improving cardiac output are relegated to avoiding anything that has the potential to enhance automaticity.

Induced hypothermia results in decreased oxygen requirements and automaticity. Electrolytes, such as magnesium, potassium, and calcium, should be monitored frequently and maintained at their upper limits of normal. The use of catecholamines should be avoided, as should sedation or paralytic agents that are sympathomimetics. Atrial or dual-chambered pacing can be used to provide AV synchrony. Although digoxin was used to improve contractility in the past, Walsh et al [25] reported no demonstrable value in a study of 71 children with postoperative JET.

The popularity and success of IV amiodarone makes it an attractive pharmacologic agent for use in patients with postoperative JET. Beta blockers should be avoided because of their negative inotropic effects. IV amiodarone is the pharmacologic treatment method of choice if the previously discussed maneuvers fail to improve hemodynamics.

## Nursing implications

The critical care nurse is pivotal in the assessment and recognition of JET after surgery for CHD. As a result of constant ECG surveillance, the bedside nurse is generally the first to note the electrical changes associated with JET [23]. These changes should be documented with ECG rhythm strips at regular intervals, and the child's physician should be notified at once.

Patients with JET after surgery for CHD should be kept well sedated, medicinally paralyzed, and minimally stimulated. Families of patients with post-operative JET are generally anxious as a result of the cardiac surgery, and if extubation efforts have been initiated, they may become more anxious and confused when the process is reversed. Critical care nurses in the intensive care unit should explain carefully the arrhythmia in terms the family can understand, the clinical interventions that may be undertaken, and the arrhythmia's transient nature. The importance of controlling the arrhythmia early also should be stressed.

## Ventricular tachycardia in infants and patients with congenital long QT syndrome

Ventricular tachycardia in children is defined as three or more repetitive excitations that originate from the ventricles at a rate 10% faster than sinus rhythm [26]. It is a relatively uncommon tachy-arrhythmia in children and accounts for less than 20% of arrhythmias in children [26]. The most worrisome ventricular tachyarrhythmias occur in very young pediatric patients and patients with congenital LQTS.

### Incessant ventricular tachycardia in very young patients

Ventricular tachycardia in infancy and childhood without structural heart disease is a relatively rare event [27]. In contrast to adults, one possible cause in very young patients (defined as younger than 5 years of age) [28] is that of a cardiac tumor or myocardial hamartoma. These tumors may be located inside or outside of the myocardium. Once the arrhythmia is controlled medically, surgically, or both, it generally regresses, which makes long-term treatment no longer necessary [28]. Rapid ventricular rates often compromise stroke volume and cardiac output and may lead to pulseless ventricular tachycardia or ventricular fibrillation.

### Electrocardiographic characteristics

The ECG characteristics for ventricular tachycardia can be found in Table 2. In most infants with ventricular tachycardia secondary to a cardiac tumor, the ventricular rate could be as slow as 132 bpm and as fast as 300 bpm [28]. In rare cases, the rate could exceed 300 bpm. The P wave may or may not be visible; however, if it is visible, it can either appear behind each QRS complex, which indicates retrograde conduction, or be completely dissociated from the QRS complex at a rate slower than the ventricular rate (Fig. 6). The QRS morphology is different from that of sinus rhythm, although it may not always be prolonged in duration for age according to age-specific guidelines [26].

### Clinical interventions

According to pediatric advanced life support guidelines [1], the treatment method of choice for hemodynamically unstable ventricular tachycardia is direct current, synchronized cardioversion starting at a dosage of 0.5 to 1 J/kg body weight. Sedation is desirable, but cardioversion should not be delayed to establish vascular access. If readily available, a

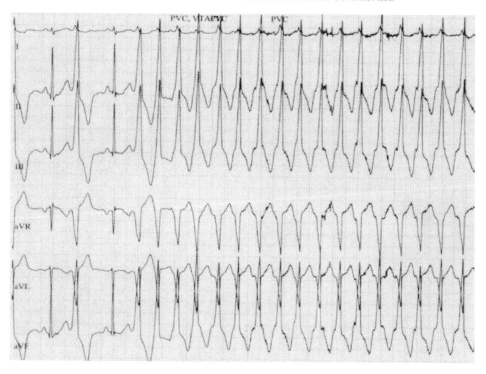

Fig. 6. Simultaneous 6-lead ECG recording in a patient who experienced ventricular tachycardia. Note the difference in QRS morphology from the first and third complexes and the remainder of the recording.

12-lead ECG should be obtained. If three attempts at cardioversion are not successful, anti-arrhythmic drug therapy should be initiated using amiodarone, procainamide, or lidocaine. These patients occasionally require inotropic support to help maintain adequate cardiac output and blood pressure.

Because of a long history of success with terminating ventricular arrhythmias, lidocaine should be used first, followed by amiodarone if the QT interval is believed to be normal. If amiodarone is not available, procainamide is a viable option. Lidocaine is a Class Ib anti-arrhythmic agent that is well known for its anesthetic effects. It is a sodium channel blocker that actually increases the (ventricular) fibrillation threshold [29] but on rare occasions can be pro-arrhythmic.

*Nursing implications*

When administering continuous IV lidocaine, the infusion site should be monitored frequently for vein irritation. A child's mental status should be assessed for any drug-related changes, such as somnolence, confusion, paresthesias, or seizures. Newborns may be more sensitive to changes in level of consciousness because the half-life of lidocaine is slightly prolonged compared with other children (ie, 3 hours compared with 2 hours) [19].

Critical care nurses should document the response to all clinical interventions. Families of young children with ventricular tachycardia need psychosocial support from their health care providers and explanations of their child's condition and treatment options in terms that they can understand. Brief, simple, and frequent explanations are of great benefit to parents and primary caregivers.

*Ventricular tachycardia in patients with congenital long QT syndrome*

Congenital LQTS is a genetic disorder in which the QT interval is prolonged. It is a familial cardiac electrical repolarization disorder in which ion channel function is altered [30]. This alteration in ion channels prolongs the action potential and results in a propensity for ventricular tachycardia and sudden cardiac death (Fig. 7). The type of ventricular tachycardia associated with congenital LQTS is known as torsades de pointes, which is a rare form of polymorphic ventricular tachycardia. It is charac-

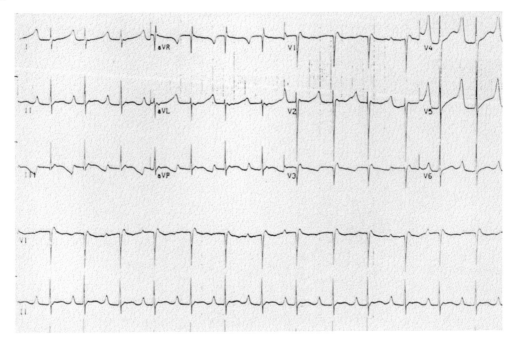

Fig. 7. A 12-lead ECG with rhythm strip in a child with a prolonged QT interval.

terized by QRS complexes that "twist" around a center axis [31]. In addition to being associated with LQTS, torsades de pointes also can be caused by type Ia anti-arrhythmic drugs (eg, procainamide, quinidine, and disopyramide), type III agents (eg, sotalol and amiodarone), and tricyclic antidepressants [9].

*Electrocardiographic characteristics*

The ECG characteristics of ventricular tachycardia can be found in Table 2. Torsades de pointes is characterized by QRS changes in amplitude (height) and polarity, which resemble a "twisting of the points" (Fig. 8).

*Clinical interventions*

Because of difficulty synchronizing to the QRS complex in polymorphic ventricular tachycardia, the initial treatment method for torsades de pointes is

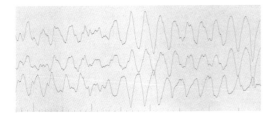

Fig. 8. Surface ECG leads I, II, and III in a patient with torsades de pointes.

external defibrillation at 2 J/kg body weight followed by 4 J if a second attempt is needed [9]. Beginning with lidocaine, pharmacologic agents should follow if cardioversion is not successful. Magnesium sulfate (Table 2) is a useful secondary agent and can be administered simultaneously with lidocaine. Pacing at a slightly increased rate also may help to stabilize patients. Amiodarone or procainamide should not be administered to patients with LQTS because each can cause further QT prolongation. Esmolol also has been used successfully in ventricular tachycardia associated with LQTS [32]. Long-term therapy for patients with LQTS includes the placement of an implanted cardioverter defibrillator.

*Nursing implications*

Nursing implications for the child who experiences torsades de pointes are essentially those previously described for incessant ventricular tachycardia in very young patients. A major difference in patients with LQTS is that certain events may trigger their episodes of tachycardia (eg, emotional stress, loud noises, and physical exertion). These event triggers require major changes in a child's lifestyle [33]. There are numerous medications that patients with LQTS should avoid, a list of which can be found on the Website for the University of Arizona's Center for Education and Research on Therapeutics [34]. Some of the more common medications to be avoided include erythromycin and its derivatives, ketoconazole and its derivatives, and tricyclic antidepressants.

If a child is newly diagnosed, there is much patient and family education to be imparted. Topics include not only an overview of the pathophysiology of the disease but also activity restrictions, possible treatment modalities, and drugs to be avoided. All family members are encouraged to become trained in basic life support; some families opt to obtain external automated defibrillators [9].

## Bradyarrhythmias

The most common cause of bradycardia in children is hypoxia, which in most cases responds to improvements in oxygenation. Bradycardia can cause shock from inadequate cardiac output, whether sinus bradycardia or AV block. Two primary bradyarrhythmias that are rarely seen in adults are likely to result in hemodynamic compromise in children: (1) sinus node dysfunction as a result of surgery for CHD and (2) congenital complete atrioventricular block.

### Sinus node dysfunction

The broad phenomenon of sinus node dysfunction, also referred to as sick sinus syndrome, consists

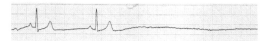

Fig. 10. Sinus arrest in a patient after surgery for an atrial septal defect.

of a wide array of bradyarrhythmias, including sinus bradycardia (Fig. 9), sinus pause/arrest (Fig. 10), sinoatrial exit block, slow escape rhythm (including junctional bradycardia), and the bradycardia-tachycardia (brady-tachy) syndrome. The primary cause of sinus node dysfunction is atrial surgery for CHD, and the most common manifestations in children include sinus bradycardia, junctional bradycardia, and the brady-tachy syndrome [5].

### Electrocardiographic characteristics

The ECG characteristics of sinus node dysfunction vary according to which arrhythmias are present. Sinus bradycardia is exhibited by a slow sinus rate (for age) with low amplitude P waves. The QRS complexes are narrow, unless bundle branch block is present. In junctional bradycardia, the ECG characteristics are the same as sinus bradycardia, with the exception of P waves, which are generally absent. In the brady-tachy syndrome, sinus or junctional bradycardia alternates with episodes of IART.

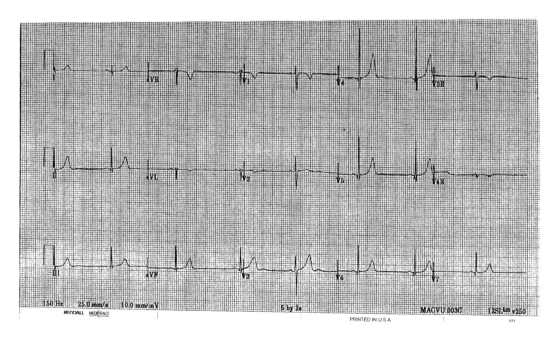

Fig. 9. A 15-lead ECG in patient with sinus bradycardia. The P waves are small in amplitude.

*Clinical interventions*

Atropine is the initial treatment method of choice for bradyarrhythmias secondary to sinus node dysfunction in children after surgery for CHD. It is an anticholinergic agent that can be used for symptomatic bradycardia; however, it must be administered at the recommended dosage (Table 2) to provide a dose large enough to produce the desired effect yet not small enough to cause a paradoxic decrease in heart rate. It is fairly long-acting (ie, 45 minutes to 1 hour) and usually results in an increase in the sinus rate.

If atropine is not successful in providing an adequate heart rate, isoproterenol is the next pharmacologic agent of choice. Isoproterenol is a beta-adrenergic agonist that is used for patients with hemodynamically unstable bradycardia (sinus or AV block) that is resistant to atropine [1]. It also has vasodilatory and positive inotropic effects.

If atropine or isoproterenol does not provide a rate fast enough to promote adequate perfusion, transcutaneous or transvenous temporary pacing should be instituted. If this bradyarrhythmia occurs in the immediate postoperative period, epicardial pacing wires can be used for temporary pacing.

*Nursing implications*

The nurse who cares for children with bradycardia and hemodynamic compromise should provide airway support, ensure adequate oxygenation and ventilation, and correct any other underlying causes [1]. Transcutaneous pacing is painful for children and if this intervention is successful, sedation is necessary. Nurses who care for children who require temporary pacing with any approach should be knowledgeable concerning the implications associated with each approach and possess the ability to assess pacemaker function. [9]

*Congenital complete atrioventricular block*

Congenital complete atrioventricular block is a relatively rare occurring bradyarrhythmia with an estimated prevalence of 1 in 15,000 to 1 in 20,000 live births [35]. It is associated with maternal connective tissue disorders and the presence of CHD. In utero diagnosis is commonly made by 20 and 30 weeks' gestation because of fetal bradycardia or a history of maternal connective tissue disorder [36]. Hemodynamic stability depends totally on the ventricular rate and cardiac anatomy. In the presence of CHD,

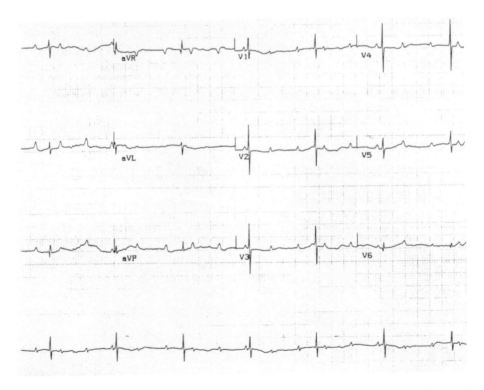

Fig. 11. A 12-lead ECG recording with rhythm strip in an infant with complete AV block. There is complete AV dissociation with an atrial rate that is approximately 2.5 times the ventricular rate.

this bradyarrhythmia may be more likely to result in hemodynamic compromise. In some cases, a fetus develops hydrops fetalis, which may prompt early delivery by cesarean section and immediate intervention with temporary or permanent pacing.

*Electrocardiographic characteristics*

The ECG characteristics of congenital complete atrioventricular block can be found in Table 2. In patients with congenital complete atrioventricular block, there is absolutely no electrical communication between the atria and ventricles (Fig. 11). The atrial and ventricular rates are regular with a slower ventricular rate.

*Clinical interventions*

Immediate clinical interventions for the neonate, infant, or child who exhibits severe symptoms related to congenital complete atrioventricular block (eg, hydrops fetalis, congestive heart failure, or low cardiac output) include support inotropic agents and temporary pacing while awaiting placement of a permanent cardiac pacemaker [9]. Although the indications vary, most pediatric cardiologists would agree that a ventricular rate less than 50 to 55 bpm or less than 70 bpm in the presence of CHD is an indication for pacemaker implantation [37]. Pharmacologic agents that are helpful in this situation include atropine and isoproterenol, as discussed in the previous section. Temporary pacing could be accomplished transcutaneously or transvenously.

*Nursing implications*

Nurses who care for children with congenital complete atrioventricular block who experience hemodynamic instability have the responsibility of providing advanced life support. In many cases, the diagnosis has been made in utero. The birth is controlled, and an effort by the obstetric, neonatal, and pediatric cardiovascular teams provides timely pacemaker implantation. If using temporary transcutaneous pacing in infants, the moderate amount of skeletal muscle stimulation is likely to impair respiration, so consideration should be given to intubation and artificial ventilation [38].

**Pulseless rhythms**

Pulseless rhythms in children are relatively rare and consist of pulseless ventricular tachycardia and ventricular fibrillation. The ECG characteristics of pulseless ventricular tachycardia are the same as that for incessant ventricular tachycardia in very young patients but without a mechanical response. Because clinical interventions and nursing implications are the same for pulseless ventricular tachycardia and ventricular fibrillation, the following discussion focuses solely on the latter.

*Ventricular fibrillation*

Ventricular fibrillation is exceptionally rare in the pediatric population. It is characterized by uncoordinated ventricular activity or depolarizations that result in no contractility of the ventricles and the complete absence of cardiac output [26]. Basically, the ventricles merely quiver, which renders the heart completely nonfunctional. Ventricular fibrillation can resemble artifact (electrical interference) or asystole (ie, fine ventricular fibrillation) on the surface electrocardiogram. In addition to the various disease etiologies associated with ventricular fibrillation, it also can result from hypoxia, electrical shock, chest trauma, and hypothermia [26].

*Electrocardiographic characteristics*

The ECG characteristics of ventricular fibrillation can be found in Table 2. Basically, there are no rate, rhythm, visible P waves, and identifiable QRS complexes in ventricular fibrillation (Fig. 12).

*Clinical interventions*

Collapse rhythms require immediate initiation of cardiopulmonary resuscitation and pediatric advanced life measures, including airway support with adequate oxygenation and ventilation. Any other underlying causes should be corrected as soon as possible. Chest compressions should be given while charging the defibrillator.

Patients with ventricular fibrillation should undergo immediate defibrillation at 2 J/kg body weight as an initial dose. If a second attempt is required, the dose is increased to 2 to 4 J/kg, followed by 4 J/kg if a third attempt is needed. After three defibrillation attempts, epinephrine should be given (Table 2) and defibrillation attempted again. Other pharmacologic agents that can be used include amiodarone, lidocaine, magnesium sulfate, sodium bicarbonate, calcium chloride, and procainamide. In rare cases, emergency cardiopulmonary bypass has been used to sustain systemic circulation until the underlying cause of the ventricular fibrillation can be corrected [39].

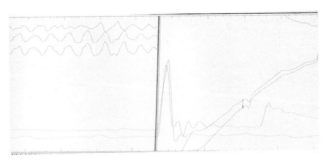

Fig. 12. Surface leads I, II, and III of a patient in the catheterization laboratory who exhibited ventricular fibrillation during implanted cardioverter defibrillator implantation. The patient was successfully defibrillated, which resulted in a ventricular paced QRS complex and resumption of adequate arterial pressure.

*Nursing implications*

Because the morphology of ventricular fibrillation is similar to that of a displaced ECG electrode, nurses first should confirm that a patient is breathless and pulseless. Prompt defibrillation should be performed using the largest paddle size possible for the child's body weight [40]. If administering IV amiodarone, it is important to monitor the child for hypotension and the ECG for bradycardia and QT interval prolongation. Nurses should provide ongoing information at frequent intervals to the child's family or, if unable to do so, should designate another health care professional or chaplain to do so.

Unfortunately, some children who experience ventricular fibrillation do not survive. In situations such as this, the nurse must be able to provide psychosocial and emotional support to the parents. Ancillary services that might be helpful to the family include the clergy, social services, and psychiatry. Parents express various emotions with the loss of a child, including, but not limited to, extreme shock, disbelief, guilt, denial, withdrawal, or avoidance. Parents should be given the opportunity to hold their child at an appropriate time after an unsuccessful resuscitation, and nurses should provide as much emotional support as possible to them at this difficult time.

**Summary**

Children with cardiac rhythm disturbances can present unique challenges to critical care nurses and other health care providers. In most cases, children remain hemodynamically stable with ample time to institute non-emergent interventions. In some cases, the arrhythmia produces hemodynamic compromise, which requires more emergent interventions. By becoming knowledgeable about cardiac arrhythmias in children and being able to identify which child's arrhythmia has the potential to impair cardiovascular hemodynamics, critical care nurses can become more confident in caring for these patients and their families.

**References**

[1] American Heart Association/Academy of Pediatrics. Textbook of pediatric advanced life support provider manual. Dallas: American Heart Association; 2002.

[2] Pearn J. Successful cardiopulmonary resuscitation outcome reviews. Resuscitation 2000;47(3):311–6.

[3] Ludomirsky A, Garson Jr A. Supraventricular tachycardia. In: Gillette PC, Garson Jr A, editors. Pediatric arrhythmias: electrophysiology and pacing. Philadelphia: WB Saunders; 1990. p. 380–426.

[4] Ko JK, Deal BJ, Strasburger JF, Benson Jr DW. Supraventricular tachycardia mechanisms and their age distribution in pediatric patients. Am J Cardiol 1992; 69(12):1028–32.

[5] LeRoy SS, Dick II M. Supraventricular arrhythmias. In: Zeigler VL, Gillette PC, editors. Practical management of pediatric cardiac arrhythmias. Armonk (NY): Futura Publishing; 2001. p. 53–109.

[6] Nadas AS, Daeschner CW, Roth A, et al. Paroxysmal tachycardia in infants and children: study of 41 cases. Pediatrics 1952;9(2):167–81.

[7] Lubbers WJ, Losekoot TG, Anderson RH, et al. Paroxysmal supraventricular tachycardia in infancy and childhood. Eur J Cardiol 1974;2(1):91–9.

[8] Fisher DJ, Gross DM, Garson A. Rapid sinus tachycardia: differentiation from supraventricular tachycardia. Am J Dis Child 1983;137(2):164–6.

[9] Knick BJ, Saul JP. Immediate arrhythmia management. In: Zeigler VL, Gillette PC, editors. Practical management of pediatric cardiac arrhythmias. Armonk (NY): Futura Publishing; 2001. p. 161–230.

[10] Burri S, Hug MI, Bauersfeld U. Efficacy and safety of intravenous amiodarone for incessant tachycardias in infants. Eur J Pediatr 2003;162(12):880–4.

[11] Celiker A, Ceviz N, Ozme S. Effectiveness and safety of intravenous amiodarone in drug-resistant tachyarrhythmias of children. Act Paediatr Jpn 1998;40(6): 567–72.

[12] Perry JC, Knilans TK, Marlow D, et al. Intravenous amiodarone for life-threatening tachyarrhythmias in children: 135 cases. J Am Coll Cardiol 1993;22(1): 95–8.

[13] Figa FH, Gow RM, Hamilton RM, et al. Clinical efficacy and safety of intravenous amiodarone in infants and children. Am J Cardiol 1994;74(6):573–7.

[14] Perry JC, Fenrich AL, Hulse JE, et al. Pediatric use of intravenous amiodarone: efficacy and safety in critically ill patients from a multicenter protocol. J Am Coll Cardiol 1996;27(5):1246–50.

[15] Walker GM, McLeod K, Brown KL, Franklin O, Goldman AP, Davis C. Extracorporeal life support as a treatment of supraventricular tachycardia in infants. Pediatr Crit Care Med 2003;4(1):52–4.

[16] Jaeggi E, Fouron JC, Drblik SP. Fetal atrial flutter: diagnosis, clinical features, treatment, and outcome. J Pediatr 1998;132(2):335–9.

[17] Lundberg A. Paroxysmal tachycardia in infancy: follow-up of 47 subjects ranging in age from 10 to 26 years. Pediatrics 1973;51(1):26–35.

[18] Garson A, Bink-Boelkens M, Hesslein PS, et al. Atrial flutter: a collaborative study of 380 cases. J Am Coll Cardiol 1985;6(4):871–8.

[19] Perry JC. Medical antiarrhythmic therapy. In: Gillette PC, Garson Jr A, editors. Clinical pediatric arrhythmias. 2nd edition. Philadelphia: WB Saunders; 1999. p. 231–48.

[20] Zeigler VL. Postoperative rhythm disturbances. Crit Care Nurs Clin North Am 1994;6(1):227–35.

[21] Fishberger SB, Wernovski G, Gentles TL, et al. Factors that influence the development of atrial flutter after the Fontan operation. J Thorac Cardiovasc Surg 1997;113: 80–6.

[22] Bink-Boelkens M, Velvis H, van der Heide JJ, et al. Dysrhythmias after atrial surgery in children. Am Heart J 1983;106(1):125–30.

[23] Zeigler VL. Cardiac rhythms in the pediatric population: supraventricular rhythms. In: Paul SC, Hebra J, editors. The nurses' guide to cardiac rhythm interpretation: implications for patient care. Philadelphia: WB Saunders; 1998. p. 205–20.

[24] Gillette PC. Diagnosis and management of postoperative junctional ectopic tachycardia [editorial]. Am Heart J 1991;118:192–4.

[25] Walsh EP, Saul JP, Sholler GF, et al. Evaluation of a staged treatment protocol for rapid automatic junctional tachycardia after operation for congenital heart disease. J Am Coll Cardiol 1997;29(5):1046–53.

[26] Garson Jr A. Ventricular arrhythmias. In: Gillette PC, Garson Jr A, editors. Pediatric arrhythmias: electrophysiology and pacing. Philadelphia: WB Saunders; 1990. p. 427–500.

[27] Pfammatter JP, Paul T. Idiopathic ventricular tachycardia in infancy and childhood: a multicenter study on clinical profile and outcome. Working Group on Dysrhythmias and Electrophysiology of the Association for European Pediatric Cardiology. J Am Coll Cardiol 1999;33(7):2067–72.

[28] Zeigler VL, Gillette PC, Crawford Jr FA, et al. New approaches to treatment of incessant ventricular tachycardia in the very young. J Am Coll Cardiol 1990;16(3):681–5.

[29] Reder RF, Rosen MR. Basic electrophysiologic principles: application to treatment of dysrhythmias. In: Gillette PC, Garson Jr A, editors. Pediatric cardiac dysrhythmias. New York: Grune and Stratton; 1981. p. 121–43.

[30] Vincent GM. The molecular genetics of the long QT syndrome: genes causing fainting and sudden death. Annu Rev Med 1998;49:263–74.

[31] Hayes DL, Maue-Dickson W, Stanton MS. Dictionary of cardiac pacing: electrophysiology and arrhythmias. Miami Lakes: Peritus Corporation; 1993.

[32] Balcells J, Rodriguez M, Pujol M, et al. Successful treatment of long QT syndrome-induced ventricular tachycardia with esmolol. Pediatr Cardiol 2004;25(2): 160–2.

[33] Zeigler VL, Gillette PC. Ventricular arrhythmias. In: Zeigler VL, Gillette PC, editors. Practical management of pediatric cardiac arrhythmias. Armonk (NY): Futura Publishing; 2001. p. 111–60.

[34] Center for Education and Research on Therapeutics, University of Arizona. Drug lists QT. Available at: http://www.qtdrugs.org/medical-pros/drug-lists/drug-lists.htm. Accessed June 15, 2004.

[35] Michäelsson M, Jonzon A, Riesenfeld T. Isolated congenital complete atrioventricular block in adult life: a prospective study. Circulation 1995;92(3):442–9.

[36] Buyon JP, Hiebert P, Cope J, et al. Autoimmune-associated congenital heart block: demographics, mortality, morbidity, and recurrence rates obtained from a national neonatal lupus registry. J Am Coll Cardiol 1998;31(7):1658–66.

[37] Gregoratos G, Cheitlan MD, Conill A, et al. ACC/AHA guidelines for implantation of cardiac pacemakers and antiarrhythmia devices. J Am Coll Cardiol 1998;31(5):1175–209.

[38] Beland MJ. Noninvasive transcutaneous pacing in children. In: Birkui PJ, Trigano JA, Zoll PM, editors. Noninvasive transcutaneous cardiac pacing. Mount Kisco (NY): Futura Publishing Company; 1993. p. 91–8.

[39] Cochran JB, Tecklenburg FW, Lau YR, et al. Emergency cardiopulmonary bypass for cardiac arrest refractory to pediatric advanced life support. Pediatr Emerg Care 1999;15(1):30–2.

[40] Atkins DL, Sirna S, Kieso R, et al. Pediatric defibrillation: importance of paddle size in determining transthoracic impedence. Pediatrics 1988;82(6):914–8.

ELSEVIER
SAUNDERS

Crit Care Nurs Clin N Am 17 (2005) 97 – 102

CRITICAL CARE
NURSING CLINICS
OF NORTH AMERICA

# The Role of Thermoregulation in Cardiac Resuscitation

## Marie Lasater, RN, MSN, CCRN*

*Neurosurgery Intensive Care Unit, Barnes Jewish Hospital, One Barnes-Jewish Plaza, St. Louis, MO 63110, USA*

For the past three decades, measures to mitigate permanent brain damage associated with cardiac arrest have been investigated. As patients were being admitted into the first intensive care units in the late 1960s, it became evident that focusing resuscitation efforts solely on the heart left many patients with neurologic compromise, if they even survived to hospital discharge. Permanent brain damage associated with cardiac arrest is multifactorial, but three predominant factors, which potentially can be modified, are (1) duration of arrest (no-flow time), (2) duration of cardiopulmonary resuscitation (low-flow time), and (3) body temperature. This article explains the impact of thermoregulation in a cardiac arrest survivor and describes timely nursing measures that promote neuroprotection through the achievement of optimal patient temperature.

## Physiologic mechanisms of thermoregulation

Body temperature is maintained by a balance between metabolic heat production and passive heat loss by several mechanisms. Nursing measures can used to regulate body temperature by modulating metabolic and passive means.

### Metabolic heat production

The hypothalamus is the body's thermostat, and it regulates heat production and heat loss. The body produces heat from metabolic processes and through exercise with the skeletal muscles. When the body is too cool, as per the preset hypothalamic thermostat that always strives to maintain homeostasis close to the optimal human temperature of 37°C or 98.6°F, several mechanisms are put into play. For short-term heat production, the hypothalamus is responsible for skin vasoconstriction, which inhibits evaporative, and conductive heat loss and piloerection, which inhibits convective and radiative heat loss. The hypothalamus also causes an increase in heat production by causing shivering, which produces heat by shaking of the skeletal muscles.

### Mechanisms for heat loss

The body uses three main mechanisms for heat loss, also mediated by the hypothalamus. All mechanisms discussed increase the amount of heat loss from the body by conductive, evaporative, convective, and radiative modes. In response to even a slightly elevated temperature, the hypothalamus inhibits sympathetic centers that cause vasoconstriction, which results in intense skin blood vessel dilation. This dilation can increase the rate of heat transfer to the skin as much as eightfold [1], which allows heat transfer by passive means. Sweating is also initiated, which also removes body heat. Finally, heat production mechanisms, such as the shivering response, are inhibited.

## Effect of temperature on oxyhemoglobin dissociation curve

Body temperature is one factor that affects how tightly oxygen is combined with the heme portion of hemoglobin. Normally, 97% of oxygen is carried in the body combined with hemoglobin in the red blood

* 14786 Highway 63, Licking, MO 65542.
*E-mail address:* calhorselover@yahoo.com

cells, and the rest is dissolved in the water of plasma. As body temperature rises, the oxyhemoglobin dissociation curve shifts to the right, releasing oxygen from the blood cell to the plasma and providing oxygen to meet the highly increased metabolic demands. The net effect is depletion of the oxygen supply. To understand this concept, think of a person with heat stroke and the dizziness and confusion that can accompany it. These symptoms occur in part because of lack of oxygen available to the cells. Conversely, with a decrease in body temperature, the oxyhemoglobin dissociation curve shifts to the left, "latching" onto oxygen and keeping it tightly bound to hemoglobin. Consider a person who has suffered hypothermia. The body still has plenty of oxygen molecules, but they are not available to the cells because they are bound tightly to hemoglobin. The person affected gradually becomes sleepier, a condition that may progress to coma if left untreated. This is why gradual rewarming of a victim with hypothermia is important. The technique allows blood cells to release their captured oxygen gradually to tissue cells without abruptly increasing metabolic demand, as would occur with too-rapid rewarming. Several recent studies, which are discussed in the following sections, have explored the therapeutic use of hypothermia and the neuroprotection that it affords.

## Hypothermia and neuroprotection

The exact mechanism of neuroprotection afforded via hypothermia is not known, although the benefits of even mild hypothermia have been well documented in several multicenter, randomized trials [2–5]. Researchers have demonstrated repeatedly that every 1°F reduction in brain temperature reduces the metabolic rate of brain cells by up to 10% [6]. It has been postulated that lowering of the core temperature to 34°C (93°F) may reduce cell injury by suppressing excitotoxins and free radical reactions, stabilizing cell membranes, reducing intracellular acidosis, and reducing abnormal electrical activity [7].

Although demonstration of the neuroprotective effects of hypothermia after cardiac arrest by examination of actual tissue changes in the human brain is not feasible, studies in animal models have shown a marked reduction in the number of viable neurons in normothermic, as compared with hypothermic, animals. In one animal study, hypothermia maintained for 24 hours at 34°C was shown to prevent necrotic striatal neuronal cell death after induced asphyxic cardiac arrest, and the effect was sustained for 11 days without side effects [8]. The duration of hypother-

mia also seems to be a factor in neuroprotection. Several studies concur that brief or mild hypothermia may only delay cerebral damage [6].

Although the optimal duration and degree of hypothermia have not been established, recently published studies suggest that 12 to 24 hours may be the optimal duration of hypothermia after cardiac arrest in humans and that 32° to 34°C may be the optimal hypothermic temperature for such patients [1,5,7,9–13]. Further research is clearly indicated in this area.

## Current clinical studies

Clinicians familiar with the Guidelines 2000 for Cardiopulmonary Resuscitation and Emergency Cardiovascular Care, disseminated by the American Heart Association and the International Liaison Committee on Resuscitation, already may be aware that there was no mention of induction of hypothermia after return of circulation as a strategy to improve short- and long-term outcomes. These guidelines include an algorithm for rewarming of hypothermic patients [14]. Since these guidelines were published, myriad clinical trials have provided level 1 evidence (one or more randomized clinical trials in which the lower limit of confidence interval for treatment effect exceeds the minimal clinically important benefit) that the induction of hypothermia improves functional outcome in adults.

In a 2002 published Australian study, 77 patients who were admitted unconscious after out-of-hospital cardiac arrest were randomly assigned to treatment with hypothermia (core temperature reduced to 33°C within 2 hours after return of spontaneous circulation and maintained at that temperature for 12 hours) or normothermia. The outcome measure used was survival to hospital discharge with adequate neurologic function to be discharged to home or rehabilitation. In the experimental (hypothermia) group, 49% achieved a good outcome, compared with 26% of patients in the control (normothermia) group [10]. Another multicenter study conducted in Europe, also published in 2002, enrolled 273 patients resuscitated after cardiac arrest caused by ventricular fibrillation. The primary endpoint was a favorable neurologic outcome within 6 months, secondary endpoints were mortality within 6 months, and the rate of complications within 7 days. Fifty-five percent of the patients in the hypothermia group had a favorable neurologic outcome compared with 39% of patients in the normothermia group. The mortality rate at 6 months was 41% in the hypothermia group compared with

55% in the normothermia group [2]. A third, large, multicenter study from Norway, published in 2003, was designed as an historic cohort observational study of all patients admitted to hospitals in four different regions of Norway with spontaneous circulation after out-of-hospital cardiac arrest. The study included 459 patients. Among other factors, body temperature of less than or equal to 37.8°C was identified as an in-hospital factor associated with survival [15].

## Accuracy and limitation of different temperature measuring devices

### Cranial temperature versus core temperature

Not all methods of measuring temperature are alike. The most crucial temperature reading for purposes of neuroprotection is the cranial temperature. Unless a patient has a ventricular bolt with a cranial thermistor, direct assessment of the temperature inside the brain is not possible. Brain temperatures do not exactly parallel temperatures obtained in other parts of the body, but generally cranial temperature is higher (up to 2°C) than rectal temperatures. In previously published neurologic studies, increased brain tissue injury and worsened functional outcomes were found when the brain temperature exceeded 39°C [16]. Other studies have shown that larger temperature gradients, more than 2° between brain and body, reflect brain ischemia [17]. Although cranial temperature measurement is beyond the scope of this article, it is wise for clinicians to remember that temperatures measured via other means are likely lower than a patient's cranial temperature.

### Methods and limitations of different methods of measuring body temperature

Although esophageal and bladder temperature monitoring occasionally may be used, in routine clinical practice, temperatures are measured via oral, rectal, axillae, groin, pulmonary artery, and tympanic membrane sites. All of these temperature measurement modes are acceptable, but have limitations that affect their accuracy if not properly obtained.

### Oral measurements

Oral temperatures obtained in the posterior sublingual pocket are considered fairly accurate because of close proximity to lingual and external carotid arteries. On average, oral temperature is lower than core body temperature by 0.5°C. To obtain accurate results, a patient must keep the thermometer under the tongue, breathe nasally, and refrain from talking while a reading is being taken. If the patient has taken food or fluids by mouth, smoked, or chewed gum within 15 minutes of the reading, the accuracy can be affected. There has been some debate regarding the accuracy of oral temperatures taken on orally intubated patients. It was believed that the temperature of humidified air being delivered and the inability of the patient to form a tight seal around the thermometer would result in inaccurate readings. A retrospective review of ten studies that addressed this concern indicated that in patients with a stable hemodynamic status, the posterior sublingual pocket is a valid method of obtaining body temperature in critically ill orally intubated patients [18].

### Rectal measurements

Although generally considered more accurate than oral temperatures, rectal temperatures are slower to track changing core temperatures because the rectum has no thermoreceptors. Rectal temperature measurements may be affected by the insulating effect of fecal material in the rectum and improper probe depth. Core temperature may change in the opposite direction of rectal temperature. This change occurs because heat passes from the rectum into the blood, not from blood into the rectum, which causes a lag time in temperature equilibration of up to 1 hour.

### Axillae and groin

Axillae and groin sites are popular because of their ease of use and noninvasiveness. Unfortunately, clinical accuracy of these sites is questionable. These sites are not located close to thermoreceptors and may not reflect temperature fluctuations. Readings may be as much as 2.2°F (1.2°C) lower than actual core temperature. In shock states, peripheral vasoconstriction also affects the reading. Temperature measurement via these modalities is not recommended when accuracy is imperative.

### Pulmonary artery

Measurement of temperature via a pulmonary artery catheter is considered the "gold standard" of core temperature against which all others are measured. Pulmonary artery measurements also have the advantages of providing continuous readouts of temperature data and, depending on monitoring equipment used, the ability to set alarms to alert the clinician if patient temperature exceeds preset limits. Despite their obvious advantages, pulmonary artery catheters are limited by their cost, relative complexity, and the fact that they cannot be inserted if a patient has received thrombolytic therapy after myocardial infarction because of the potential of bleeding complications.

*Tympanic measurements*

A great deal of controversy exists regarding the accuracy of tympanic temperatures. Tympanic temperatures are generally regarded to give false low readings. Despite this fact, tympanic thermometry is becoming more widespread because it is convenient, fast, and noninvasive. In theory, tympanic temperatures should have a high degree of accuracy because the tympanic membrane shares the same vascular supply as the hypothalamus. Accuracy of tympanic temperatures can be affected by several factors, however, such as cerumen in the ear. Various operator errors include not placing the infrared reader of the tympanic thermometer at the tympanic membrane, inaccurate depth of thermometer insertion, and not obtaining a tight seal. In a recent study that compared not only tympanic and oral temperature measurements but also different brands of tympanic thermometers, researchers obtained a total of 812 temperature measurements from 72 subjects. Measurement methods included oral, tympanic, and pulmonary artery catheter. Thirty-two percent of obtained measurements were from febrile patients and 68% were from afebrile patients. Researchers concluded that when used correctly, oral thermometry is the best method of temperature monitoring in critically ill patients when pulmonary artery temperatures are not available [19].

**Methods of lowering body temperature**

Body temperature can be lowered by medications, increasing heat loss by conduction and convection, and intravascular cooling methods.

*Medications*

Antipyretic agents are administered to suppress fever and lower body temperature. They generally do not have a great effect on a normothermic person. These agents fall into two main categories: (1) steroidal and (2) nonsteroidal. Although rarely used for this purpose, steroids can act as antipyretics as they block fever by inhibiting the production of endogenous pyrogens by white blood cells. Nonsteroidal anti-inflammatory drugs (eg, aspirin, indomethacin, ibuprofen, and ketorolac) are effective antipyretic medications that act in the preoptic and anterior hypothalamic region to inhibit the production

of prostaglandin $E_2$. Acetaminophen works by blocking prostaglandins that can cause fever, without anti-inflammatory effects. Acetaminophen and aspirin are the most widely used antipyretics, and although they have their own individual precautions (ie, the hepatic effects of acetaminophen and the coagulation effects of aspirin), they can be alternated safely in therapy to reduce the risk of deleterious side effects. When a patient has no access via rectal or oral means, ketorolac can be administered intravenously for effective antipyretic action [20].

*Conduction and convection loss*

Since the first nurse cared for the first febrile patient, methods to reduce fever by body heat loss via conduction and convection have been used. Tepid baths, alcohol baths, cooling blankets, and application of ice packs to the groin and axillae are all methods of increasing passive heat loss from the body. If a patient is too chilled, however, shivering results, with either an increase in body temperature or a poor response to cooling methods. A small dose of meperidine (12.5–25 mg) is an off-label but effective method of attenuating the shivering response [21]. As the beneficial effects of hypothermia become more widely known, researchers are studying other means to lower core temperature effectively. Callaway et al [22] attempted to provide significant cranial cooling by the application of ice to the heads and necks of cardiac arrest subjects. They did not find a statistically significant reduction in cranial temperature (as assessed by surrogate cranial temperature measurements via nasopharyngeal and tympanic temperatures). Hachimi-Idrissi et al [23] tested the speed and feasibility of a cooling helmet device to achieve a target temperature of 34°C in unconscious patients who suffered out-of-hospital cardiac arrest. In the study, they achieved the core temperature target 180 minutes after restoration of spontaneous circulation after arrest. They also found that lactate concentration and oxygen extraction were significantly lower in the helmet group compared with the non-helmet group.

*Intravascular temperature modulation*

Intravascular cooling techniques repeatedly have been shown to be more effective in preventing fever than the conventional methods of antipyretic medications and surface-cooling techniques previously described [16]. Bernard et al [5] studied the rapid infusion of large volume (30 mL/kg), ice cold lactated Ringer's intravenous fluid to comatose survivors of out-of-hospital cardiac arrest. After the infusion, they found a significant decrease in median core temperature from 35.5° to 33.8°C. They also found significant improvements in mean arterial blood pressure, renal function, and acid-base status. No patient developed pulmonary edema. Although commercial intravascular cooling devices are available [24], in actual clinical practice, simply placing intravenous lines so they run through an ice bath for cooling before fluids enter the patient is a gentle, clinically effective, and virtually cost-free method of intravascular cooling.

## Adverse consequences of hypothermia

Maintaining hypothermia is not completely without risk. Complications include cardiac arrhythmias, coagulation defects, pneumonia, and hypotension [25].

### Arrhythmias

The major arrhythmia seen with therapeutic hypothermia is bradycardia, which actually can be beneficial in a cardiac arrest victim because of the effect it has of reducing myocardial work. Bradycardia associated with hypothermia is refractory to atropine, because it is caused by decreased spontaneous depolarization of pacemaker cells [26].

### Coagulation defects

Coagulation time increases in severe hypothermia, which causes a delay in the clotting cascade. Cases of disseminated intravascular coagulation have been seen with cases of severe hypothermia (<33°C) but have not been reported with therapeutic hypothermia.

### Pneumonia

With severe hypothermia, a patient is also at risk for pneumonia because of decreased ciliary motility and decreased minute volume secondary to a drop in respiratory rate and decreased tidal volume. These effects can by mitigated by mechanical ventilation.

### Hypotension

Hypotension with hypothermia can be observed. This complication is secondary to many factors, including inhibition of baroreceptors and "cold diuresis," which is believed to be caused by an inhibition of antidiuretic hormone.

### Sepsis

Sepsis has been found to develop in patients with hypothermia in higher numbers than patients with normothermia. This difference has not been found to be statistically significant, but warrants further investigation [2].

## Effect of hypothermia on certain drugs used in cardiac arrest

Hypothermia can render a patient refractory to atropine. Other studies in animals have shown that vasopressin and amiodarone (cordarone) are not effective in treatment of ventricular fibrillation associated with hypothermia [27]. Because therapeutic hypothermia is used more frequently as a therapeutic modality, it is likely that many more drugs will be identified whose effects are attenuated by this therapy.

## Summary

Regulating a patient's body temperature long has been within the scope of practice of the critical care nurse. Different measures and modalities have been used to achieve normothermia in the past. Recent research has demonstrated how crucial body temperature can be, not only because of its potential for neuroprotection, but also because of its effects on all body systems. The general consensus of current literature is that maintaining mild hypothermia at 32° to 34°C for 12 to 24 hours after cardiac arrest may provide optimal neuroprotection with minimal complications for patients.

## References

[1] Guyton A. Body temperature, temperature regulation, and fever. In: Guyton A, editor. Textbook of medical physiology. 6th edition. Philadelphia: WB Saunders; 1981. p. 886–98.

[2] Hypothermia After Cardiac Arrest Study Group. Mild therapeutic hypothermia to improve the neurologic outcome after cardiac arrest. N Engl J Med 2002; 346(8):549–56.

[3] Sterz F, Holzer M, Roine R, et al. Hypothermia after cardiac arrest: a treatment that works. Curr Opin Crit Care 2003;9(3):205–10.

[4] Holzer M, Sterz F, and the Hypothermia After Cardiac Arrest Study Group. Therapeutic hypothermia after

cardiopulmonary resuscitation. Expert Rev Cardiovasc Ther 2003;1(2):317–25.

[5] Bernard S, Buist M, Monteiro O, et al. Induced hypothermia using large volume, ice-cold intravenous fluid in comatose survivors of out-of-hospital cardiac arrest: a preliminary report. Resuscitation 2003;56(1): 9–13.

[6] Schaller B, Graf R. Hypothermia and stroke: the pathophysiological background. Pathophysiology 2003; 10(1):7–35.

[7] Kabon B, Bacher A, Spiss CK. Therapeutic hypothermia. Best Pract Res Clin Anaesthesiol 2003;17(4): 551–68.

[8] Agnew D, Koehler R, Guerguerian A, et al. Hypothermia for 24 hours after asphyxic cardiac arrest in piglets provides striatal neuroprotection that is sustained 10 days after rewarming. Pediatr Res 2003; 54(2):253–62.

[9] Safar P, Behringer W, Bottiger B, et al. Cerebral resuscitation potentials for cardiac arrest. Crit Care Med 2002;30(4 Suppl):S140–4.

[10] Bernard S, Gray T, Buist M, et al. Treatment of comatose survivors of out-of-hospital cardiac arrest with induced hypothermia. N Engl J Med 2002;346(8): 557–63.

[11] Xavier LC, Kern KB. Cardiopulmonary resuscitation guidelines 2000 update: what's happened since? Curr Opin Crit Care 2003;9(3):218–21.

[12] Morris MC, Nadkarni VM. Temperature regulation after cardiac arrest...timing is everything! Crit Care Med 2003;31(2):654–5.

[13] Hoeksel R. Mild hypothermia improved neurological outcome and reduced mortality after cardiac arrest because of ventricular fibrillation. Evid Based Nurs 2002;5(4):111.

[14] The American Heart Association in collaboration with the International Liaison Committee on Resuscitation (ILCOR). Advanced challenges in resuscitation: hypothermia. Circulation 2000;102(Suppl I):I-229–32.

[15] Langhelle A, Tyvold SS, Lexow K, et al. In-hospital factors associated with improved outcome after out-of-hospital cardiac arrest: a comparison between four regions in Norway. Resuscitation 2003;56(3): 247–63.

[16] Marion DW. Controlled normothermia in neurologic intensive care. Crit Care Med 2004;32(2 Suppl):S43–5.

[17] Sakuri A, Kinoshita K, Atsumi T, et al. Relation between brain oxygen metabolism and temperature gradient between brain and bladder. Acta Neuorchir Suppl 2003;86:251–3.

[18] Fallis W. Oral measurement of temperature in orally intubated critical care patients: state-of-the-science review. Am J Crit Care 2000;9(5):334–43.

[19] Giuliano K, Giuliano A, Scott S, et al. Temperature measurement in critically ill adults: a comparison of tympanic and oral methods. Am J Crit Care 2000; 9(4):254–61.

[20] Gerhardt R, Gerhardt D. Intravenous ketorolac in the treatment of fever. Am J Emerg Med 2000;18(4): 500–1.

[21] Sessler D. Treatment: meperidine, clonidine, doxapram, ketanserin, or alfentanil abolishes short-term postoperative shivering. Can J Anaesth 2003;50(7):635–7.

[22] Callaway CW, Tadler SC, Katz LM, et al. Feasibility of external cranial cooling during out-of-hospital cardiac arrest. Resuscitation 2002;52(2):159–65.

[23] Hachimi-Idrissi S, Corne L, Ebinger G, et al. Mild hypothermia induced by a helmet device: a clinical feasibility study. Resuscitation 2001;51(3):275–81.

[24] Schmutzhard E, Engelhardt K, Beer R, et al. Safety and efficacy of a novel intravascular cooling device to control body temperature in neurologic intensive care patients: a prospective pilot study. Crit Care Med 2002; 30(11):2481–8.

[25] Olsen TS, Web UJ, Kammersgaard LP. Therapeutic hypothermia for acute stroke. Lancet Neurol 2003; 2(7):410–6.

[26] Preston B. Effect of hypothermia on systemic and organ system metabolism and function. J Surg Res 1976;20:49–63.

[27] Schwarz B, Mari P, Wagner-Berger H, et al. Neither vasopressin nor Amiodarone improve CPR outcome in an animal model of hypothermic cardiac arrest. Acta Anaesthesiol Scand 2003;47(9):1114–8.

ELSEVIER
SAUNDERS

Crit Care Nurs Clin N Am 17 (2005) 103–107

CRITICAL CARE
NURSING CLINICS
OF NORTH AMERICA

# Index

*Note:* Page numbers of article titles are in **boldface** type.

# Your *Clinics* subscription just got better!

## You can now access the FULL TEXT of this publication online at no additional cost! Activate your online subscription today and receive...

- Full text of all issues from 2002 to the present
- Photographs, tables, illustrations, and references
- Comprehensive search capabilities
- Links to MEDLINE and Elsevier journals

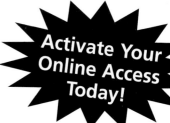

Plus, you can also sign up for E-alerts of upcoming issues or articles that interest you, and take advantage of exclusive access to bonus features!

## To activate your individual online subscription:

1. Visit our website at **www.theclinics.com**.

2. Click on "Register" at the top of the page, and follow the instructions.

3. To activate your account, you will need your subscriber account number, which you can find on your mailing label (note: the number of digits in your subscriber account number varies from six to ten digits). See the sample below where the subscriber account number has been circled.

**This is your subscriber account number**

```
*****************************************3-DIGIT 001
FEB00   J0167   C7    (123456-89)   10/00   Q: 1

J.H. DOE, MD
531 MAIN ST
CENTER CITY, NY  10001-001
```

4. That's it! Your online access to the most trusted source for clinical reviews is now available.

# theclinics.com

# Changing Your Address?

Make sure your subscription changes too! When you notify us of your new address, you can help make our job easier by including an exact copy of your Clinics label number with your old address (see illustration below.) This number identifies you to our computer system and will speed the processing of your address change. Please be sure this label number accompanies your old address and your corrected address—you can send an old Clinics label with your number on it or just copy it exactly and send it to the address listed below.

We appreciate your help in our attempt to give you continuous coverage. Thank you.

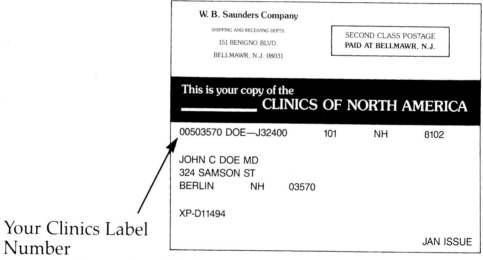

**W. B. Saunders Company**

SHIPPING AND RECEIVING DEPTS.

151 BENIGNO BLVD.

BELLMAWR, N.J. 08031

SECOND CLASS POSTAGE
PAID AT BELLMAWR, N.J.

This is your copy of the
**CLINICS OF NORTH AMERICA**

00503570 DOE—J32400          101          NH          8102

JOHN C DOE MD
324 SAMSON ST
BERLIN          NH          03570

XP-D11494

JAN ISSUE

## Your Clinics Label Number
Copy it exactly or send your label along with your address to:
**W.B. Saunders Company, Customer Service**
Orlando, FL 32887-4800
Call Toll Free 1-800-654-2452

Please allow four to six weeks for delivery of new subscriptions and for processing address changes.